Living with
Pernicious Anaemia
and Vitamin B$_{12}$ Deficiency

Living with
Pernicious Anaemia
and Vitamin B$_{12}$ Deficiency

Martyn Hooper

Foreword by
Dr Fiona Porter

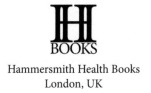

Hammersmith Health Books
London, UK

First published in 2013 by Hammersmith Health Books – an imprint of
Hammersmith Books Limited
14 Greville Street, London EC1N 8SB, UK
www.hammersmithbooks.co.uk

Whilst the advice and information in this book are believed to be true and
accurate at the date of going to press, neither the author nor the publisher
can accept any legal responsibility or liability for any errors or omissions
that may be made.

British Library Cataloguing in Publication Data: A CIP record of this book
is available from the British Library.

Print ISBN 978-1-78161-036-7
Ebook ISBN 978-1-78161-037-4

Commissioning editor: Georgina Bentliff
Designed and typeset by: Julie Bennett
Index: Dr Laurence Errington
Production: Helen Whitehorn, Pathmedia
Printed and bound by: TJ International Ltd, Cornwall, UK
Cover image: Girl Carrying a Pail by Thomas Barker of Bath © National
Museum of Wales

Contents

About the Author

Martyn Hooper founded the Pernicious Anaemia Society to provide a forum for sufferers from the condition, having suffered from vitamin B_{12} deficiency for many years without a diagnosis. To write this book – a companion to his earlier *Pernicious Anaemia: the forgotten disease* – he has drawn on the experience of the Society's 7000+ members together with classic and current research findings.

Acknowledgements

As the Chairman of the Pernicious Anaemia Society, I deal with the consequences of pernicious anaemia on a daily basis. Sufferers, and their families and friends, use various channels of communication to tell of their experiences with the condition and to seek advice. It is clear from a brief perusal of the Society's online forum, Facebook page. and the websites and Facebook pages of other patient groups, that there is a fundamental problem not only with the way in which patients obtain an accurate diagnosis and adequate treatment, but also with the efficacy of B_{12} replacement-therapy injections. It is evident that replacement-therapy does not always lead to a cessation of the many symptoms associated with pernicious anaemia and B_{12} deficiency and that often these ongoing symptoms significantly affect sufferers' private and public life. Furthermore, when things become desperate, it is the moderators of the Society's online forum who are able to dispense help and advice. I never cease to be amazed at the professionalism and knowledge of this team and I have to thank them for their dedication and commitment in dealing with what can be quite traumatic and challenging stories.

When things get really tough I am asked to intervene on a more personal basis. This involves writing letters of support, providing statements and dispensing telephone advice. Because I am in a unique position to know the full range of problems that patients experience, I took the decision to write this book, which focuses on the problems associated with patients remaining symptomatic even after their treatment has begun. Using the Society's website, online forum and Facebook pages, I requested that members of the Pernicious Anaemia Society send me their stories of how they were diagnosed and treated and how the condition affects their everyday lives. I would like to thank all of those who took the time to put pen to paper and relate their often disturbing experiences. Without these stories this book would not have been possible. The downside is that it has not been possible to use all of the material that was sent to me, simply because there was so much of it – one further indication of how widespread these problems are.

My thanks go also to the many volunteers who give their time so freely to help out in the Society's offices: Anna, Megan, Taylor, Nicole, Joanna and Danny all help to ensure that the Society does what it does so well.

Special thanks go to Carrie-Anne Carr for her tireless work in organising regional support groups and for liaising with the various bodies and institutes responsible for making healthcare decisions. Thanks also go to the other Trustees of the charity, who continue to place their faith in me, for their continued support.

Georgina Bentliff of Hammersmith Health Books has been a pillar of support and I am grateful for her advice, guidance and doing all she could to get this book published by the almost im-possible deadline set by me.

Finally, my thanks go to my wife for her continued support in everything I do. Without her, the Pernicious Anaemia Society, and the good work that it does, simply would not exist.

Foreword

When I first started working as a general practitioner in a Welsh Valley practice, I thought that I knew everything I needed to know about pernicious anaemia: you make your diagnosis, then give B_{12} injections. Simple! To my surprise, some patients were unhappy and it became evident that this simple condition was not simple at all. I decided to take the lead in my practice, drawing up a workable protocol, and getting my partners to refer all their pernicious anaemia patients to me.

I began experiencing vague health symptoms myself, which I was unable to fathom. You can imagine my shock when I myself was diagnosed with pernicious anaemia. How had I missed this? Wasn't I an expert? And why wasn't my treatment working? When an invitation to a Pernicious Anaemia Society symposium arrived in my mail, I thought it would be a good idea to learn more.

This was the first time I met Martyn. I shall never forget that day. The symposium was poorly attended by the medical profession. I shrank down in my seat as I listened to the horrifying experiences that patients were having: the delayed diagnoses; the difficulties in persuading GPs to provide treatment; the ongoing symptoms.

Martyn talked about his own experiences, and I was inspired by his determination to help other sufferers. Here was a man, with no medical background, who knew more about pernicious anaemia than I did! I drew from his knowledge that day, and have continued to do so in the years since.

This book is a great opportunity for everyone to gain some of his insight. Martyn has shared his own story, and also those of other Pernicious Anaemia Society members. He has highlighted not only how the disease affects patients, but how it impacts on their family and friends. He has drawn from both his own experiences, and his many years as Chairman of the Pernicious Anaemia Society, and given a precise account of where the NHS falls short of good condition management. For patients, it will help alleviate the feeling of isolation that is felt by many sufferers.

I honestly believe that most GPs (like myself a few years back) fall into the 'It's a simple condition with a simple treatment' approach. For these doctors, the book will highlight the broad spectrum of the condition and more appropriate treatment options.

Martyn is to be commended for bringing pernicious anaemia to the forefront of the health agenda, and this book is a great guide for doctors and patients alike. Raising awareness of the condition, how it is diagnosed and how it is treated, will hopefully lead to a long overdue review by the medical profession, and a set of guidelines that best reflect how pernicious anaemia should be managed in the 21st century.

Dr Fiona Porter
General Practitioner

Introduction

In May 2002 I was finally told the reason why my legs were totally numb and wouldn't work properly. I had developed pernicious anaemia. It had crept up on me over what was probably a number of years. It was responsible for my breathlessness, sudden mood swings, erratic behaviour, memory loss, confusion, continual tiredness and exhaustion and would eventually mean that I would have to take early retirement from lecturing in further and higher education.

For years I had attributed the tiredness and mental symptoms to my age – I had just turned 40 – and only visited my doctor when my legs became numb and I started walking with an unusual gait. Even then it took a year for me to get a diagnosis, during which time I suffered quite severe nerve damage to my spinal cord. In the end, it was only because my sister, who is a nurse, decided to take a blood sample that I found out the cause of my problems – a lack of vitamin B_{12}.

When I was told that my problems were all due to my lacking a simple, readily available vitamin (it's found in all animal products such as milk, fish, meat and eggs), I believed that the time it had taken to receive a diagnosis was a fluke, a one-off, and my experience was exceptional. In an age where medical advances have made accurate and quick diagnoses the norm, surely my experience was the result of unhappy circumstances. I wanted to find out more about my disease and started searching the internet. This was in the age before broadband connections and Google and it took a long time before I realised that there simply wasn't any patient information to be had.

When I was forced into early retirement I decided that I would establish a webpage that would contain a fact sheet explaining in plain English the nature of the disease to newly diagnosed patients. I thought, wrongly, that I knew all there was to know about the disease and with this in mind I set about setting up the website which would let newly diagnosed patients download a leaflet explaining the nature of the disease. I sent out a mass email aimed at web designers asking for some help in setting up a charity (although at this time I had no intention of creating a charity – but saying I would simplified things) and received a reply from a designer in North Wales. He stated that he was just setting up his own business as a web designer and had always promised himself that he would choose one charity to help for free, so he was offering to help. I travelled to North Wales to meet with him and over lunch explained what was needed. He suggested that the best solution would be to set up an online forum where patients could not only find information about their condition, but could also interact with one another and provide peer support. By the time I had travelled back to South Wales the forum was live.

Within days it became glaringly obvious from reading people's stories about their experiences that there were serious problems, not only with the time it was taking for patients to be told the reason why they felt so poorly, but also with the way in which their pernicious anaemia was being treated. I was genuinely surprised; I had thought that my own experience in waiting over two years for a diagnosis was unique. The postings on the forum told a different story and it soon became clear that somebody needed to bring these problems to the attention of the medical community. So, that is how the Pernicious Anaemia Society started and that is what it is still doing – raising awareness of the problems that patients are faced with in getting diagnosed quickly and treated adequately.

People who have pernicious anaemia lack the essential vitamin B_{12} which is needed for healthy red blood cells. In the middle of the 1920s, it was discovered that people with pernicious anaemia could be kept alive by giving them large amounts of raw liver to eat. Before then. people who were diagnosed as having pernicious anaemia would die a slow death (see account in chapter 6, page 110) – hence the 'pernicious' tag. In the late 1940s, scientists produced artificial vitamin B_{12} which could be injected into a patient's muscle and therefore correct the deficiency. Note that this was not a cure, but it was a therapy which would, or rather should, stop patients with the disease from dying. Doctors had now made the pernicious aspect of the disease redundant and, as long as the sufferer was diagnosed quickly there should be no reason to suppose that he or she would not be able to live a normal life. The consequence of the disease, the lack of vitamin B_{12}, would be corrected.

However, as the online forum revealed right from the very beginning, many sufferers, me included, still experience some or all of the symptoms of the deficiency *after* the replacement therapy has begun. More bizarrely, some patients can be severely deficient in the vitamin and yet will display none of the symptoms; the deficiency is picked up by chance only when investigating some other complaint. Why some people with pernicious anaemia still experience symptoms of B_{12} deficiency even after that deficiency appears to have been rectified has not been explained. If there is one thing that the Pernicious Anaemia Society can be proud of, it's the fact that people who complain of the symptoms after treatment has been started now no longer have to be satisfied with their physician's explanation that he or she is imagining them and that once the replacement therapy injections have begun then all will be well. Likewise, it has not been explained why some patients will have experienced none of the symptoms in the run-up to their diagnosis.

Before the Pernicious Anaemia Society came into existence there was no vectoring point where people with the disease could easily interact with other sufferers and share experiences. Individuals who reported back to their doctor that they were still experiencing symptoms even though they were having replacement therapy injections thought they were alone in this. When the physician ran another blood test to explore why the injections were not working and the test invariably showed normal or above normal levels of vitamin B$_{12}$, patients would have no basis on which to argue that they were not imagining the symptoms or refuse when then offered anti-depressants to ease what the physician would believe to be the patient's anxiety. This chain of events still happens, but the sheer number of members of the Society who do not see some or all of their symptoms disappear after their injections have started means that not everyone can be imagining that they are still suffering from the effects of vitamin B$_{12}$ deficiency. Many of these Society members have to make changes to their lifestyle that can and do affect deeply family life, social life and careers. What is missing is the scientific explanation as to why the symptoms of vitamin B$_{12}$ deficiency do not magically disappear once replacement therapy has begun, although there are plenty of clinical scientists who are aware of the problem.

This book has several purposes. It seeks to raise awareness among medical professionals and sufferers (along with their families and friends) that a great many people with pernicious anaemia will still experience the symptoms of vitamin B$_{12}$ deficiency after they have started to receive treatment to correct the deficiency. It also seeks to make sufferers aware that they may have to make changes to their lifestyle to some extent to cope with the still present symptoms, and, in some cases, those changes will be drastic. I also hope that, by drawing on patients' experiences in developing different ways of dealing with their condition, that this will help others with the disease to deal with their problems better and to live as normal a life as possible.

There is a further reason for writing this book. As I said earlier, one of the worst aspects of having pernicious anaemia and still being symptomatic is that in most cases doctors will tell the patient that he or she is imagining the symptoms, as any blood test will show above average levels of B_{12} in the patient's blood. This in itself leads to the patient being confused and even doubting his or her own experiences. What makes this much worse is when the sufferer's family sides with the doctor and wrongly believes that the sufferer is imagining his or her symptoms. This then leads to family members refusing to make any adjustments to everyday life and brings with it a myriad of associated problems, including labelling the patient as lazy, anti-social, a hypochondriac and many other negative descriptions. Hopefully this book will allow family members to understand that the sufferer is not imagining his or her symptoms and this in turn will encourage the family to understand the problems associated with pernicious anaemia and be more sympathetic.

As I mentioned above, before the Pernicious Anaemia Society came into being, there was no community where patients and sufferers could relate their experiences, tell of their symptoms and compare treatments. Because there was no such forum, individual doctors could not be blamed for believing that once treatment had started, patients' symptoms would disappear; all the medical textbooks told them this was so and patients' blood results would support this belief. What the Pernicious Anaemia Society has unwittingly done is to bring to doctors' attention the fact that patients are having problems getting diagnosed and once diagnosed do not necessarily become symptom free. As Chairman of the Pernicious Anaemia Society, which has over 7500 members, I am only too aware of how the problems with the diagnosis, and treatment, of pernicious anaemia are affecting people's everyday lives.

This book is intended as a companion to my earlier book, *Pernicious Anaemia: the forgotten disease*, which concentrates more on the nature of the disease and how it is diagnosed and treated. For the past seven years I have been in a unique position to collect case studies of members' experiences and a small number of these case studies are to be found in this book – one of which I also included in my previous publication as it demonstrates so well the problems faced by sufferers. Some of them tell harrowing tales of negligence and missed opportunities. Others tell of marital strife, career changes and poor quality of life. There are tales of sadness and woe and they are about people of all ages and race. However, these case studies are just a few of many thousands of similar experiences; a quick trawl through the Pernicious Anaemia Society's online forum or the many Facebook pages relating to B_{12} deficiency and pernicious anaemia will soon reveal similar stories.

As well as people's experiences of poor diagnosis and treatment I have also been made aware of serious problems with the techniques used to diagnose B_{12} deficiency in general, and pernicious anaemia in particular. Whilst it is easy to understand that these failings in the current diagnostic procedures are unfair to patients suffering from B_{12} deficiency, it has to be realised that they are also letting medical practitioners down as doctors are being misled by false data that is being used to make a diagnosis. I will explain these problems later (see chapter 6).

When I first started the Pernicious Anaemia Society and began to become aware of the problems with patients not receiving an early and accurate diagnosis, and often not receiving treatment according to their needs, I was naïve enough to think that all I needed to do was to tell a few medical professionals what I had uncovered and the problems would soon be put right. Seven years later we, as a Society, after a great deal of hard work and being faced with setbacks that are too many to recall, have recently had some success in making those responsible for making decisions relating to health aware of these problems. I have, after many years of struggling to climb what was, at times, a very greasy pole, finally made it into the offices of key players in the UK's health system. Doors are opening and at last I, as a representative of a patient support group that has over 7,500 members, am able to provide health professionals with evidence that there are problems with the diagnosis and treatment of pernicious anaemia. In addition (although I find myself whispering this), there is some evidence that change is on the way. Now is the time to reveal just how these problems with the current way in which pernicious anaemia is diagnosed and treated affect sufferers' lives. And I want everyone to know about this – sufferers, their family members, their friends, employers and medical professionals. This book is all about the *impact* pernicious anaemia has on people's lives; about the impact of poor diagnostic procedures and often inadequate treatment. And remember, there is no cure for pernicious anaemia. It can be treated but, as yet, there is still no cure.

Chapter 1

What is pernicious anaemia?

It was 7 December 1908 and, from his home in Durham in the UK, a recently bereaved husband wrote to his cousin:

My Dear Cousin,

I have to thank you for your kind letter of sympathy with me in the loss of my dear wife. She has been ailing for over a year, suffering from what the doctors call "Pernicious Anaemia", and it seems to be a disease which is almost impossible to cure.

She managed to get to Silloth in the middle of summer and got a little better at first, but soon fell away again and grew gradually weaker.

Jon has not seen her since Uncle Tom's funeral at Silloth. I think I will be through at Oulton[i] occasionally, and when the days get a little longer I will take the opportunity to call on you some time.

I am

Yours sincerely

Rich[d] Birkett

i A village in Cumbria

The note is written in beautiful copper-plate writing on a small card folded in the middle. The front of the card has a black border that immediately identifies it as being associated with a recent death.

The note is interesting because it tells us that Mr Birkett's poor wife had been diagnosed with pernicious anaemia, which was 'impossible to cure' and that the patient had been suffering from the disease for over a year. Over one hundred years after Mr Birkett set about writing to his relatives thanking them for their messages of condolence, doctors still have no cure for pernicious anaemia.

Although there is no cure, people no longer routinely die of the condition. Once it has been diagnosed, remedial treatment is available. The problem is the treatment is often inadequate and life from then on is dominated by the tension between receiving the right treatment, leading as normal a life as possible, and dealing with the expectations of family, friends, employers and colleagues that diagnosis and treatment mean being symptom free. This is what this book is about – living with B$_{12}$ deficiency in general and pernicious anaemia in particular.

What is pernicious anaemia?

Anaemia is defined in dictionaries as 'blood deficiency' and a good medical dictionary describes over 90 different types of anaemia, usually defined according to their cause. By far the commonest, and the most well known, is iron-deficient anaemia. Here the sufferer will be lacking in the essential mineral iron, which could be due to blood loss, and will therefore not be able to produce **haemoglobin**, the red substance in our blood that is responsible for carrying oxygen to all the cells in our body and carbon dioxide away from them. Haemoglobin is transported around the body in our red blood cells. It is therefore essential that we have the right number of these and that they are healthy. If we lack sufficient red blood cells, then the same thing happens – oxygen is unable to be taken to wherever it is needed, which is just about everywhere. So, in order to have healthy blood you need decent levels of iron (to make the haemoglobin) and healthy levels of red blood cells (to transport the haemoglobin).

If you have pernicious anaemia, this means you have a problem with your red blood cells – they will be faulty and will not last very long and may, in some cases, be enlarged and a strange shape as well (see page 105). Put another way, if you have pernicious anaemia your red blood cells will, one way or another, be rubbish.

So why are some people deficient in vitamin B_{12}? B_{12} is an essential vitamin that we cannot make ourselves, so you may be thinking it is because these people do not get enough B_{12} in their diet. However, B_{12} is found in *all* animal products, including fish, shellfish, meat and dairy produce. Some animal products, such as liver, contain very high amounts of the vitamin but don't give it up as readily as others; B_{12} is more 'bio-available' in dairy products. Vegans and vegetarians *are* therefore at risk of developing vitamin B_{12} deficiency if they exclude all animal products from their diet. However, most vegetarians and vegans are aware of this risk and take vitamin supplements in a variety of ways to ensure that they do not develop any deficiency. In addition, some foods, including most breakfast cereals, have vitamin B_{12} added to them along with many other vitamins and minerals with which they are 'fortified'. This means a normal healthy person eating a balanced non-vegan diet will find it quite difficult to become deficient in vitamin B_{12}. A 'balanced diet', by the way, is not to be confused with the current 'five a day' campaign to encourage us all to eat five portions of fruit or vegetables a day. A balanced diet also contains fish, meat or dairy produce – there is no B_{12} in fruit and vegetables. It therefore follows that a person who eats a balanced diet will only become deficient in vitamin

B$_{12}$ if he or she has a problem in absorbing the vitamin from the food that he or she has eaten.

Absorbing vitamin B$_{12}$

The whole human digestive process begins when you pop something into your mouth. As you chew the food it mixes with chemicals in your saliva to form what is known as 'bolus'. When you swallow this it travels down the 'oesophagus' and into your stomach, where the main process of digestion begins. The stomach churns the bolus into 'chyme' (think of this as a sort of soup, though you may prefer not to). Lurking in the lining of part of the stomach (called the 'fundus') are some very important cells called the 'parietal cells'. These produce two essential things – gastric acid[ii] and 'intrinsic factor'. Intrinsic factor is a protein that is responsible for absorbing B$_{12}$ from any food that contains it, but it doesn't do it yet; it just hangs around waiting for the gastric acid to do its bit in the digestive process by going to work on the chyme. The partially digested chyme is then pushed through to the small intestine. So, by this stage, the food has been mixed with saliva, when it was chewed, and with gastric acid and intrinsic factor in the stomach.

The small intestine[iii] has three separate parts. First the chime enters the 'duodenum', where proteins in the chime are broken down and any iron that is in the food is absorbed. It is then pushed into the 'jejunum' where most of the nutrients in the food are absorbed into the bloodstream. Then it travels to the final part of the small intestine – the 'ileum'. It is in the ileum that the intrinsic factor (that was produced back in the stomach and

---

ii Gastric acid is a mixture of hydrochloric acid, potassium chloride and sodium chloride. The stomach also produces bicarbonate to neutralise the worst effects of too much hydrochloric acid.
iii Also called the small bowel.

has simply been carried along through the first two parts of the small intestine) binds with any vitamin B_{12}. This intrinsic factor can only bind to food containing B_{12} – if the food (such as fruit) contains no B_{12}, then obviously no B_{12} can be extracted and the intrinsic factor will have been produced for no reason. If you can think of no other reason to eat some fish or cheese or meat, do so, so that the intrinsic factor your stomach is producing (if you are healthy) has something to do.

Special cells that line the wall of the ileum then recognise the B_{12}/intrinsic factor compound and it is through these cells that the B_{12} is absorbed into the bloodstream via a complex series of chemical reactions. Once in the bloodstream the B_{12} then goes about the business of building healthy red blood cells.

Now, all of this highly complex biological process occurs when you eat or drink anything – or rather it should. If the process goes wrong at any stage, for any reason, vitamin B_{12} deficiency will result. For people with pernicious anaemia the problem will be with the intrinsic factor. It may be they cannot produce any (or enough) because the parietal cells in the stomach lining are not working properly, due to an antibody that destroys these cells. Alternatively, they may produce the intrinsic factor but then, and for reasons that doctors still don't understand, produce antibodies that destroy the intrinsic factor. These are called 'intrinsic factor antibodies' or, more correctly, 'anti-intrinsic factor antibodies'. When a disease is caused by the body essentially turning on itself it is called an 'auto-immune disease'. So pernicious anaemia is, in most cases, an auto-immune disease.[iv]

This is what makes pernicious anaemia different from other anaemias; no matter how much food containing B_{12} is eaten, the sufferer won't be able to extract the vitamin because he or she will lack the intrinsic factor needed to absorb it into the bloodstream.

iv Other auto-immune diseases include type 1 diabetes, Hashimoto's thyroiditis and psoriasis, to name but three of a long list.

And the reason he or she will not have any intrinsic factor is because he or she is either not producing any, or producing it but also producing an antibody that destroys it.

Producing intrinsic factor also becomes a problem for older people. As we age, the lining of our stomach begins to waste away – doctors say it suffers from atrophy. Gastric atrophy becomes more common with advancing age and leads to many digestive problems, including not producing intrinsic factor. This is why pernicious anaemia is often (wrongly) seen as a disease that affects only the elderly, but in this case it is not classic auto-immune pernicious anaemia by deficiency due to gastic atrophy.

There is one further group of people who will also have problems in absorbing vitamin B$_{12}$. As I described earlier, vitamin B$_{12}$ enters the bloodstream in the part of the small intestine called the ileum. Some people are unfortunate enough to have had to have their ileum surgically removed for one or more of several reasons (an ileostomy). It stands to reason that those people will lack this piece of apparatus that is essential for absorbing B$_{12}$ and will not therefore have healthy red blood cells. This group of patients will also need replacement B$_{12}$ therapy for life, though they can produce intrinsic factor, but whether they have pernicious anaemia is a matter for discussion, as is whether people with gastric atrophy do. Is it only patients with an auto-immune problem who can be classed as having pernicious anaemia? Whatever the cause, if you cannot absorb vitamin B$_{12}$ from food one thing is certain – you'll experience the same symptoms.

Symptoms of B$_{12}$ deficiency

As I have explained, people with pernicious anaemia will be unable to extract vitamin B$_{12}$ from food and will consequently become deficient in this essential vitamin. This will mean that their red blood cells won't work properly in transporting oxygen around the body. But what will the sufferer experience as a result, and how will he or she feel?

Well, before we go into the list of symptoms of B_{12} deficiency we need to be aware of a number of problems that are encountered when dealing with the end results of vitamin B_{12} deficiency. The first of these is that some people will have what doctors would consider to be adequate amounts of B_{12} in their blood but will experience many of the symptoms of the deficiency, while on the other hand, there are people who will have extremely low amounts of B_{12} in their blood and yet will have none of the symptoms. Why is this? As far as I've been able to discover nobody has thoroughly investigated this phenomenon, but I believe it is because of three issues.

Issue 1: what is a 'normal' level of vitamin B_{12}?

Firstly, it could be that the current threshold for determining whether a person is deficient in B_{12} is far too low. There is currently a very lively and healthy debate amongst medical professionals as to what this threshold should be. Writing in late 2011, Professor David Smith and Professor Helga Refsum said:

> We believe that the traditional cut-off value of 148 pmol/l[v] is too low. We suggest that physicians should consider treating patients who show symptoms but have vitamin B_{12} levels above this value, particularly those in the low-normal range up to approximately 300 pmol/l, to see whether their symptoms are relieved.[1]

---

v 'pmol/l' stands for picomoles per litre. A 'mole' is a measurement used in chemistry to describe the amount of a substance rather than its volume or weight. A picomole is one trillionth (10^{12}) of a mole. October 23rd has been named as mole day by North American chemists, but how it is celebrated I haven't been able to discover – perhaps it's left up to each individual scientist to choose how to make that day special. What is certain is that the festivities begin at 6:02 am and end at 6:02 pm.

This would mean that patients who experience the symptoms of B_{12} deficiency but who have B_{12} levels above the threshold that is used currently to determine deficiency would receive replacement therapy B_{12} and this could and should relieve their symptoms. As things stand at the moment, sufferers who experience the symptoms of B_{12} deficiency but whose blood level of B_{12} is above – and sometimes only just above – the level currently used to define a deficiency will remain untreated, or be treated for something else.

Interestingly, some doctors today don't bother with the results of any test that patients have had to determine whether they are deficient in B_{12}. They treat their charges according to their symptoms and not according to the results of a test that is seriously flawed (as we shall see).

Issue 2: is all B_{12} 'biologically active'?

This leads us to the second problem with diagnosis when patients have all of the symptoms but their blood results suggest that they are not deficient. The test that is currently used to determine the amount of B_{12} in a patient's blood may need to be replaced. It is called the 'competitive-binding luminescence assay', or CBLA for short, which has replaced tests based on microbiologic and radioisotope-dilution assays. Still with me? An assay is a laboratory procedure that measures the quality or quantity of something, which in this case is vitamin B_{12} (the 'analyte'). As I have already mentioned, we know that some scientists are critical of the way in which the *quantity* of the B_{12} is measured; there are others who believe the *quality* of the B_{12} that is measured is also flawed. This is because the current test doesn't distinguish between 'biologically active' B_{12} and the B_{12} that plays no part in the complex biochemical process that produces healthy red blood cells.

Biologically active B_{12} is more properly known as 'holotranscobalamin' or 'holoTC', and a new test that distinguishes between a patient's 'active' and 'inactive' B_{12} has been developed by Axis-Shield Diagnostics and is quietly being introduced into some laboratories in the UK and the USA. Astonishingly, between 70% and 90% of the B_{12} in your blood will be inactive. So, if say, the threshold for determining B_{12} deficiency is 200 pmol/l and your B_{12} level was 250 pmol/l, then you would not be considered to be deficient in the vitamin; but if only 20% of the B_{12} was found to be 'active', then the amount of B_{12} doing its bit in producing healthy red blood cells would be a worryingly low 50 pmol/l. At the time of writing there are discussions taking place on the merits of replacing the current CBLA test with the new active B_{12} test. However, the new test is not without its critics; one commentator has noted that: 'Without answers to the many important, unaddressed questions, holoTC remains an inadequately explored enigma, and assigning it primacy in clinical diagnosis is premature.'[2] This is an example of what scientists call a 'healthy debate'.

Issue 3: False negatives

The third issue that could explain why some people with apparently healthy levels of B_{12} in their blood experience the symptoms of B_{12} deficiency could be that the current test is unreliable. In fact, some believe it to be next to useless in determining the B_{12} status of patients. The CBLA has been found to give false normal readings in 22%, 26% and 35% of patients' B_{12} levels, with these figures relating to different models produced by three different manufacturers. This means that, depending on the machine used to calculate the level of B_{12} in a patient's blood, between 22% and 35% of patients were told that the status of B_{12} in their blood was at a healthy level when it wasn't.[3] The authors of the report (Carmel and Agrawal) also discovered that the test to investigate whether the patient had intrinsic factor antibodies (the auto-immune response that would effectively destroy any intrinsic factor that had been produced) was giving false normal results in 33% to 53% of cases. This means that between 33% and 53% of patients who were tested to investigate whether they had intrinsic factor antibodies were told that they didn't have them when in fact they did. That would explain why, when I was tested for intrinsic factor antibodies to explain my B$_{12}$ deficiency, the results came back as negative twice before finally proving that I did have the antibody.

Another piece of research from 2013 was also scathing about the current test. It found that machines from four different manufacturers gave false high results for B$_{12}$ status. For those interested in the detail, these were:

Elecsys E170 Cbl assay (Roche Diagnostics Corp, Indianapolis, IN, USA):
    184 pmol/l (Reference range 140 – 500).

UniCelR DxI 800 Cbl assay (Beckman Coulter, Brea, CA, USA):
    1116 pmol/l (Reference range 130 – 700)

Architect 8000i Cbl assay (Abbott Laboratories, IL, USA):
    298 pmol/l (Reference range 170 – 600)

Immulite XPi Cbl assay (Siemens Healthcare Diagnostics, Tarrytown, NY, USA):
    620 pmol/l (Reference range 142 – 725)

In all of the above, the B$_{12}$ level of the patients' blood was above the lower threshold used to determine B$_{12}$ deficiency, whereas this blood was actually deficient in the vitamin. The chemistry involved in this experiment was far too complex for me but the authors concluded:

In the meantime, (until a new and more accurate test is developed and introduced) we strongly advocate using holotranscobalamin or metabolic tests such as **homocysteine** *or* **methylmalonic acid** *(MMA) in patients with high suspicion for pernicious anaemia without a low Cbl [cobalamine] level.*[4]

The evidence therefore suggests that current tests are next to useless in determining B_{12} levels accurately and detecting any intrinsic factor antibodies. These problems could explain why 43.6% of patients with pernicious anaemia were originally diagnosed as having some other disease or medical condition before receiving an accurate diagnosis. It could also explain why 55% of members of the Pernicious Anaemia Society waited two years or more for a diagnosis, whilst 14% had to wait five years or more to be told that they had vitamin B_{12} deficiency and that the lack of that vitamin was the cause for their ill-health.[5]

In the United Kingdom, the National External Quality Assessment Service (NEQAS) is responsible for ensuring that laboratory test results are 'accurate, reliable and comparable wherever they are produced'. The problems with the current test to evaluate B_{12} status have not gone unnoticed by the service. Aware of the serious and irreversible nerve damage that can be caused by low B_{12}, the NEQAS advised in early 2013 that patients who were symptomatic of B_{12} deficiency but whose serum B_{12} was 'normal' should be treated regardless of what their blood test showed:

UK NEQAS Haematinics is keen to publicise their concerns on problems with current B_{12} assays which may be vulnerable to interference resulting in normal values despite severe cobalamin deficiency. The Committee advises that where there is a discordance between the clinical features of neuropathy such as parasthesiae, loss of joint position sense, or megaloblastic anaemia and a 'normal' B_{12} result, clinicians are advised to request *storage of serum for further testing and are advised to treat the patient with B$_{12}$ replacement therapy.*[6]

Alternative tests

There are alternative methods of identifying B$_{12}$ deficiency, including tests that measure the patient's methylmalonic acid (MMA) and homocysteine levels. The biochemistry of these tests need not concern us here (thankfully, as it is really complicated and clever stuff), but doctors are able to identify patients' B$_{12}$ status by evaluating their MMA and homocysteine, both of which will be raised if the individual has low B$_{12}$. In fact, these tests seem to be more reliable than any of the other tests used to identify any deficiency in B$_{12}$ and are universally acknowledged to be far better indicators of B$_{12}$ status than the current serum B$_{12}$ test. Given that, why aren't they used more than they are? Well, at the time of writing I am unable to answer that question. It could be either because the failings of the current test are not as yet that widely known or because doctors, while being aware of the limitations of the current test, do not fully appreciate the awful consequences of false negatives. I hope with this book it will be possible to change that awareness and reverse the current lack of urgency to correct the problems that the current test is causing. The sufferers' stories told here demonstrate the urgent need to address the failings of the current test.

Janet's story

Like many pernicious anaemia sufferers, with hindsight I had PA for a number of years before I received my first jab, but things really started to kick off on my son's seventh birthday, just after Christmas 2008. I had a run of bad colds in the run-up to Christmas but was just starting to feel better and thought I might make the pantomime we had booked to celebrate his birthday. On the morning of his birthday, however, I woke at 6 am and could not even roll over. I thought I had pulled a back muscle, but my husband called out the doctor and it turned out I had pneumonia and pleurisy. An ambulance trip and a day in hospital replaced my family trip to the pantomime.

The next few months I did not exactly feel myself but I was told it might take time to recover from the pneumonia and pleurisy, so I tried not to worry. After a few months I tried to start running again. I like to keep fit and every year used the Race for Life as a motivator to get my running shoes on. My first run of the year went well and I felt the usual exhilaration, for a few hours at least. Then it felt like I had hit a brick wall. I had never known tiredness like it, except perhaps the early days of pregnancy. Over the next few months the pattern continued – every time I exerted myself my tiredness was overwhelming and eventually the feeling just never left me. Not great when you have two young children, your own business to run and a marriage to keep happy!

In addition, my 'tummy troubles', as our family have christened them, worsened and I developed really bad eczema – something that runs in my family but had never troubled me. I had had to make mad dashes to the loo with debilitating diarrhoea at regular intervals since my son was a baby. I was pretty sure it was food related and thought I might be lactose intolerant. After a particular nasty and embarrassing bout of sickness in a National Trust car park, followed by diarrhoea, my husband forced me to go to the doctor, who gave me some strong anti-acids to settle my stomach. My stomach did improve, but my diarrhoea did not. Eventually a friend persuaded me to take a health food shop food intolerance test. Though I was very sceptical initially, I found as long as I stayed away from the foods they identified – garlic, onion, red wine and cow-dairy – I was fine. Now it seemed if I ate anything out of the ordinary my inside would be upset. It was really getting me down, so I forced myself to see my doctor.

My regular doctor was off, but the replacement was so nice that, after relating all my health worries, I broke down and cried. Not my finest hour, but I was genuinely scared. I was so tired I could not think straight, I was shouting at my children, having to have a rest after getting them to school and an afternoon nap before picking them up, just so I could cope with the few hours before they went to bed. My business was suffering, but I was so relieved that I worked for myself as if I had still been in employment I don't know what I would have done.

Thankfully the doctor was very thorough, and did a host of blood tests as well as a test for depression. I practically shouted at her that I knew I was not depressed. I knew the only thing getting me down was my physical health, but I duly completed it and she crossed it off her list. She sent me to specialists for my skin and for my digestion. She also handed me a leaflet on ME and pernicious anaemia, with the words, 'I'm pretty sure it is ME, but you do have the pernicious anaemia antibody in your system. That means you're likely to develop it in the future so you may like to read this. Your B$_{12}$ levels are low, but on the normal scale so it's nothing to worry about for now.'

I took the leaflets home and read them avidly. I certainly ticked many of the symptom boxes for both, but the 'sudden and uncontrollable bouts of diarrhoea' symptom on the pernicious anaemia sheet struck a chord, so I visited the Pernicious Anaemia Society's website. It was there I read more about the levels of B$_{12}$ and thought, I need to get a B$_{12}$ jab. 'How am I going to persuade my doctor?' I thought as I read the case histories of some people's challenge to get diagnosed. Luckily, when I saw the gastroenterologist he commented on my 'fairly low' B$_{12}$ levels, and armed with my newfound knowledge I asked, 'Do you think it would help to get some B$_{12}$ jabs?' 'Well, it's worth a go,' was his response, and he put that recommendation on his note to my doctor.

The GP read that sceptically and said she would prescribe three monthly injections for a few months to 'see how you get on, you don't need a loading dose.' Naturally, I felt better almost immediately. I could think clearly for the first time in ages, I had a bit of energy, I stopped shouting at the children. I could have wept! After a few weeks, though, I was counting the days until my next injection – something I was going to have to do for some time.

Chapter 1

Thanks to knowledge gained from the Pernicious Anaemia Society (PASOC) I realised I was one of those people who could not cope with a three-monthly injection regime, but the nurses at my practice were completely oblivious to this and could be quite brutal in their rejection of my request for a jab before my three months were up. Armed with information from Pernicious Anaemia Society I persuaded the doctor to allow me to have my jabs every two months, but still some nurses were reluctant to help and if I turned up a week before that two-month deadline I could be turned away.

I now go directly to the GP and have five-weekly jabs, though I am sure he is still not convinced that they are necessary. I get comments such as, 'Well, I must say you are looking very well,' as if I am making it up. I am a positive person and refuse to go around moping and dragging my feet, but that does not mean they don't feel like lead! In fact it is my feet and legs that have finally made me realise that I just can't even continue on this regime.

I have just had to return to the doctors to get a jab after a gap of just three weeks. During those three weeks I have pushed against my feeling of tiredness and had a lovely four days in London. Lovely, that is, apart from the fact that by the end of it my feet were burning with hot pain, all the muscles in my feet and legs were cramping and random shooting pains along the soles of my feet would take my breath away. After a week of rest nothing seemed to improve so I shared this information with my doctor. My feet have been an issue on and off for a while now and he did mention tarsal tunnel. Feeling very flat last week I looked it up and the symptoms certainly sound familiar, as do those for Grierson-Gopalan syndrome.

Even a day after having my jab the heaviness in my legs has gone and my feet feel much better. And for me this is the final push I need. I feel as though even this five-weekly regime is not working for me and I am concerned about the damage I may be doing to my body by not having enough B$_{12}$ in my system. I have been nervous about heading down the B$_{12}$ infusion route, but my fear in not having it is now greater. I would say wish me luck, but I don't feel like I need luck as I know I have the Pernicious Anaemia Society behind me every step of the way. It is no exaggeration to say I don't know what kind of state I'd be in if I hadn't found them!

So what is being done about this?

It seems clear that the way in which vitamin B$_{12}$ deficiency in general, and pernicious anaemia in particular, is diagnosed (and treated) is flawed, and there are plenty of medical professionals who know this to be the case. So why, you may ask, isn't anything being done about this? Well, there are things happening. If you remember, I said in my introduction that when I first uncovered problems with the diagnosis and treatment of pernicious anaemia I naïvely believed that as soon as I made doctors aware of this then things would change. I was naïve for four reasons – and these help to explain why nothing seems to be happening.

Firstly, health provision is an enormous sector of the economies of countries in the developed world. When one sector accounts for such a large proportion of a nation's activity, things do not change quickly – usually. Yes, the test for B$_{12}$ deficiency is flawed, but simply labelling very expensive machines redundant will not happen overnight, especially as the results of the poor diagnostic procedures do not result in death.

This leads me to my second point. The tests for B$_{12}$ deficiency and pernicious anaemia may be flawed; they may result in people waiting a long time to be told the reason why they feel so ill; but the delay and false negatives do not result in fatalities – although we don't know this for certain.

Thirdly, I believe that whilst there has been some suspicion among medical professionals that the test is far from satisfactory, it was not until the Pernicious Anaemia Society came along that it became clear that people are indeed suffering unnecessarily for many years before being diagnosed as having a deficiency in vitamin B_{12}. That's why I've been busy getting our research out there and meeting with decision makers in healthcare.

Finally, it was only in 2012 that the research was published that proved that the current test is flawed. Without that research I only had anecdotal evidence to back up my concerns.

Conclusion

Already we can see that there are serious issues with the way in which B_{12} deficiency is diagnosed and further problems with determining whether that deficiency is caused by pernicious anaemia. Whilst doctors and other medical professionals may be aware that the current test for B_{12} is far from perfect, it seems that they are not aware of the impact this is having on individual sufferers and their families and friends. What I am trying to do is raise awareness of just how these problems affect people's lives.

Chapter 2

How does pernicious anaemia affect people? The symptoms of pernicious anaemia and B$_{12}$ deficiency

How does pernicious anaemia affect people? There are some very strange issues relating to its symptoms, and perhaps the strangest of them all is something I started to discuss in chapter 1 – some people will have extremely low levels of vitamin B$_{12}$ and yet have none of the symptoms while others will experience all of the symptoms and yet when tested will be shown to have a B$_{12}$ blood level above the threshold used to diagnose deficiency. Above all, it is very important to recognise that many patients with PA still experience some or all of their symptoms to some extent or other after treatment has been started. Just why this is so hasn't been explained, but it is a fact. This is complicated by the problem that most doctors believe that once the B$_{12}$ deficiency has been rectified then the patient's symptoms *should* disappear. When their patients report that they are still symptomatic the doctor will often believe the patient is imagining the symptoms and this often leads to the patient being offered some form of anti-depressant. At the same time, it is good to remember that some patients who have full-blown, or 'classic', pernicious anaemia, and a very low level of B$_{12}$ in their blood, will often experience the symptoms only very slightly, if at all.

Sufferers who are still symptomatic after their treatment has begun are quite justified therefore in believing that the treatment that they are receiving is not working; they share this problem with many other sufferers. This could be because either the injections are not strong enough or they are not given often enough. Sometimes the patient will feel an immediate improvement in their well-being after their first injection whilst others will not feel any benefit even after many visits to the nurse. Again, nobody is able to offer a reasonable explanation for this that is based on scientific evidence. What *is* known is that sufferers who have received treatment and feel much better for it will have the same amount of B_{12} in their blood as sufferers who feel no improvement in their well-being. Faced with this problem, and no research findings to explain it, it is not surprising that doctors and the friends and family of patients consider these ongoing symptoms to be 'all in the mind'.

Not all in the mind

There are four reasons why I believe that patients who are still symptomatic after receiving treatment are *not* imagining their malaise.

Sheer force of numbers

First, there are far too many of them! Persistent symptoms and the need for more frequent injections remain by far the most common causes of complaint by members to the Pernicious Anaemia Society and the subject of a vast number of posts on the Society's online forum, as well as other social media, including Facebook. They *could*, I suppose, *all* be imagining their symptoms, but this is, I believe, highly unlikely given the vast numbers of patients involved.

Painful injections

Secondly, those injections can be very unpleasant and often hurt. Why then would sufferers want more of something that can be unpleasant unless it was for a good reason?

Top tip

The method of delivery used by most nurses is to inject the serum into a muscle – usually the patient's biceps, which are found in the upper arm. Unfortunately, some nurses are not as skilled or careful as others and how painful or painless the injections are is something of a lottery. One way in which the injection can be made less painful is if the ampoule containing the injection is allowed to come to room temperature before being broken and the contents transferred to a syringe. The injection is stored in a refrigerator and when cold is much thicker than at room temperature. Gently rolling the ampoule in your hand will soon improve its viscosity.

Enough is enough

Thirdly, patients who are lucky enough to receive injections as and when they require them (and this is the usual case outside the NHS in the UK) will no longer pester their doctor for more frequent injections and will report an improvement in how they feel. They may be receiving replacement therapy injections every 11 weeks, or every 10, 9, 8, 7, 6, 5 4, or 3 weeks – until they will finally arrive at a frequency regime that suits them; then they stop pestering their doctor. Just how many hours of doctors' time are taken up by patients making repeat visits to their GP asking for more frequent injections is unknown, but it is bound to run into many thousands every year. Some doctors will happily sanction a more frequent treatment regimen, but these tend to be the exception rather than the rule. When I was still getting injections from a nurse I was lasting about three and a half weeks before the strange tiredness (see page 26) and confusion returned.

Not just the sufferer that notices the symptoms

Finally, and perhaps the most compelling indication that sufferers are not simply imagining that they need another injection before their 12 weeks are up, is that sometimes it is not the sufferer who demands more B_{12} from their doctor, but another family member who will have noticed a deterioration in some aspect of the sufferer's behaviour. He or she may have noticed the sufferer struggling to find the right word during conversations; or starting to stumble again or becoming angry and frustrated, with changes in personality. If it is someone else asking for additional injections, it is highly unlikely the sufferers are imagining a return of his or her symptoms, or that the family is.

Medical mystery

There is something else that adds to all of this confusion. Sometimes a patient will try to find a treatment regime that suits him or her and be injecting three or four times a *day* and still not find any relief from the symptoms of B_{12} deficiency. It doesn't make sense because at the other end of the scale are patients who manage perfectly well on an injection every three months and find their symptoms never return.

I've questioned several eminent clinical researchers about this phenomenon and all have suggested that the answer lies in the mystery surrounding how vitamin B_{12} actually enters our cells. Astonishingly, as far as I have been able to discover, nobody has ever come up with an explanation as to what exactly happens with B_{12} absorption at cell level. Thankfully, one of the members of the Pernicious Anaemia Society is a highly reputable microbiologist who is currently working on this.

Topping up B_{12}

What do patients do when they require more frequent injections than those prescribed by their doctor? Well, it depends on two things: how much money they have and where they live in the world. In the UK, injectable B_{12} is only available on prescription. This is because the British Medicines Act of 1968 states that anything injectable has to be available only on prescription. In most other parts of the world it is also available over the counter at pharmacies. Where this is the case, patients who feel their symptoms returning after a period of time simply go to their pharmacy and purchase vials of B_{12} and either inject themselves or get a family member or friend to do so. This isn't ideal as the injections should be given into a muscle, which is tricky to do yourself, and the injection should be administered by somebody who has been trained to give them. And then there are the added problems of ensuring the injection site is clean and the used syringe is disposed of correctly in a lockable sharps bin. A great many members of the Pernicious Anaemia Society stock up on supplies of injectable B_{12} when on holiday in mainland Europe, where they find it hard to believe that what is so hard to get hold of in the UK is available for the equivalent of about 50p.

Then there is the internet with its online pharmacies. Yes, that's where many patients get extra supplies of the injection. It's easy, quick, cheap and potentially very dangerous and I strongly advise against buying injections this way. That it is undesirable doesn't mean, however, that this doesn't happen.

Others who have more disposable income opt to get treated outside the NHS in the UK and visit private doctors who are not only happy to inject patients however often they want, but also provide intravenous infusions of a particular form of B_{12} known as 'methylcobalamin'. Prices vary from around £100 to £600 for a consultation and an armful of B_{12}. It is these infusions that are so popular with 'celebrities' some of whom have a weekly fix of B_{12} and sometimes other vitamins.

Bill's story

Bill is 89 years old and was diagnosed as having pernicious anaemia when he was 50. Bill was a navigator in the RAF during the Second World War and completed his tour of duty (40 successful missions) during 1944–45. After being de-mobbed he became a mathematics lecturer at two colleges of further education and retired when he was 65, but kept working part-time until he was 68. Every three months, Bill visits his local doctors' surgery and receives an injection of hydroxocobalamin B_{12}. After four weeks Bill then visits a private doctor and receives another injection of hydroxocobalamin and, after another four weeks, goes back to the private doctor to receive another injection. Four weeks after that he re-visits his own surgery for his prescribed 12-weekly injection. Bill cannot function on an injection every 12 weeks and so he pays to get the more frequent replacement therapy. I asked him how much the private doctor charged him. He told me it cost him £120 for each injection which he pays for using his life savings. The cost of the ampoule of hydroxocobalamin is around 50p.

All of this needs to be seen against the background that some doctors practising in the NHS *do* sanction and prescribe an injection regime based on the needs of the patient. However, those who do so run the risk of being disciplined by the controlling health boards. When I was first diagnosed I was lucky to have a GP who would treat me according to my needs, which, as

I have said, was around every three weeks. I was lucky, and even luckier to have a sister who was a nurse and could save my time and the surgery's time by injecting me at home.

Alternative delivery methods – are injections best?

There is a growing market for alternative delivery methods for B_{12}. As we have seen, people with pernicious anaemia are unable to absorb B_{12} from food and so have to rely on injections to deliver B_{12} directly into the bloodstream. But there are alternative methods for delivering the B_{12}, including the following:

Oral tablets of cyanocobalamin: Logically these shouldn't work but strangely do raise the amount of B_{12} in blood. However, where tablets have replaced injections as the standard replacement therapy, doctors have often reverted back to the injections, finding that their patients much prefer them. This is what is currently happening in Canada. Why most patients prefer what can be a painful injection to simply taking a tablet can only be explained if the injections work whilst tablets don't – which flies in the face of established research.[7] I'm one of those sufferers who don't trust tablets as a form of replacement therapy for my B_{12} deficiency. I don't want to stop injecting myself for two reasons: firstly, because the tablets shouldn't work (I don't have any intrinsic factor to cling to the B_{12} in the tablet); secondly, I don't want to take the chance – I can still remember how I felt before I was eventually diagnosed, how I couldn't think properly or walk, and I'm not risking going back there again.

Sub-lingual sprays: These work by delivering methylcobalamin under the tongue, where it is absorbed into the bloodstream via a mucous membrane. Sub-lingual lozenges and drops work in the same way.

Skin patches: Here the B_{12} is absorbed into the bloodstream by permeating the skin.

Nasal drops and sprays: Here the B_{12} travels through a membrane in the nose into the bloodstream.

Nebulisers: Here the B_{12} is turned into a fine mist that is inhaled and, presumably, gets into the bloodstream via the lungs.

Other methods: Some people already use B_{12} tablets as suppositories and some even put drops of B_{12} into the urethra (there's a mucous membrane on the inside – we'll leave it at that).[8] In fact research carried out in the 1960 demonstrated that using anal suppositories of B_{12} is an effective way of elevating serum B_{12} levels.[9]

Whilst all of these alternative treatment therapies are growing in popularity (especially among those patients who cannot access more frequent injections than they currently receive), nobody has evaluated how effective they are. And there is the rub – how do you define *efficacy*? Any evaluation could not be based on how effective the treatment was in raising B_{12} levels; it would have to centre on how effectively the delivery method alleviated the symptoms of B_{12} deficiency experienced by individual sufferers.

The common symptoms of B_{12} deficiency

A further problem for people with B_{12} deficiency is a discrepancy between what most doctors consider to be the symptoms of this condition and the symptoms recognised by patients. The following are the somewhat vague symptoms that doctors recognise as indicators of B$_{12}$ deficiency together with the more specific description of the symptoms experienced and reported by patients. The percentage figures are taken from a survey of members of the Pernicious Anaemia Society over an 18-month period when over 1,200 members responded to a questionnaire specially designed by a practising doctor (who is a member of the Society). Results were analysed by a statistician and another practising doctor.

Tiredness versus 'the strange tiredness'

Whilst 'tiredness' is the symptom that is by far the most commonly described and experienced symptom by patients (95.5%), and is recognised as a symptom of B$_{12}$ deficiency by doctors, it goes only part of the way to describing how sufferers really feel. The tiredness of B$_{12}$ deficiency never really leaves you, and it is a tiredness that is quite specific in its effect. This is why Society members refer to it more accurately as 'the strange tiredness'. This description of the constant fatigue experienced by patients is more accurate because it distinguishes between the 'normal' tiredness experienced by ordinary people who may have been over-exerting themselves in one way or another, and the quite specific tiredness that pernicious anaemia sufferes experience, which never really goes away. Another more specific description of the tiredness experienced by people with B$_{12}$ deficiency is 'waking up tired' (87.1%), which relates to the continual, incessant fatigue experienced by sufferers. Both the strange tiredness and waking up tired are much more specific indicators than the normally attributable tiredness recognised as a symptom by doctors. Both these terms were coined and first described by members of the Pernicious Anaemia Society, who participated in an online focus group organised by the charity.

Shortage of breath versus 'the sighs'

The second most common symptom that people with B_{12} deficiency experience, and one which most doctors are aware of, is 'shortage of breath' (72.7%). However, most sufferers do not spend their day panting as if they had just run a half-marathon. Shortage of breath is a very vague term that doesn't accurately describe the problems sufferers face as they continually try to compensate for the lack of healthy oxygen-carrying red blood cells. What is happening is that because not enough oxygen is being transported through the arteries to be deposited where it is needed, the sufferer's brain automatically instructs him or her to take in more air. It doesn't matter how much air he or she ingests, there will not be a corresponding increase in the oxygen in his or her blood without healthy red blood cells to take it up, but the brain still instinctively calls for more oxygen to be inhaled. However, this doesn't usually result in the sufferer panting. The Society's online survey produced a much more specific description; namely, 'the sighs'. Instead of panting, the sufferer will usually start to take deep breaths and yawn which, when breathing out, sounds just like he or she is sighing. Once you are aware of this you become conscious of just how many sufferers go about their daily business sighing, sometimes quite loudly. 'The sighs' are a much more specific symptom than the usually quoted 'shortage of breath'.

Before we leave this symptom, it's worth noting that one of the members of the Pernicious Anaemia Society is running a sponsored half-marathon for the Society, though it is beyond most members to comprehend how he can do this.

A swollen, 'beefy', enlarged and cracked red tongue ('glossitis')

Though not as common as previously thought, the appearance of an enlarged tongue that might also be sore is a good indicator of B$_{12}$ deficiency. Around 33% of respondents to the survey had experienced this. Glossitis is also why dental surgeons are sometimes responsible for alerting people to the possibility that they may have B$_{12}$ deficiency. I know when I have gone too long without an injection because the tip of my tongue becomes quite sore.

Less widely recognised symptoms

Then there are symptoms of B$_{12}$ deficiency that are not widely recognised by medical professionals as being indicators of pernicious anaemia.

Diarrhoea

The first doctor to describe pernicious anaemia reported that the patient suffered from diarrhoea,[10] which is an experience shared by a great many members of the Pernicious Anaemia Society: nearly 57.6% reported that they experienced sudden and unaccountable bouts of diarrhoea, with 40.2% experiencing this after a bout of constipation. Strangely though, it isn't widely recognised as an early indicator of B$_{12}$ deficiency by medical professionals despite these sudden bouts of diarrhoea being so common. Many members of the Pernicious Anaemia Society were originally diagnosed as suffering from irritable bowel syndrome or Crohn's disease on their journey to eventually receiving an accurate diagnosis. When you remember that pernicious anaemia is caused by a malfunction in the digestive process it shouldn't come as a surprise that sudden bouts of diarrhoea are associated with the disease.

'The fogs'

The second of these less recognised symptoms is the inability to think clearly. Known as 'the fogs' by sufferers, this leads to the patient being unable to understand properly what is being said. Often it means that the sufferer will keep asking the same question, be unable to find the correct word for an everyday object or person, have to read and re-read passages of text in books and not remember the plot or even the outcome of a film. The fogs can last a few minutes, hours or days. I know that before I received what I consider to be adequate treatment for my deficiency, I often used to spend two or even three days of every week experiencing the fogs. And it shouldn't come as any surprise that the documentary produced by the Society in 2011 was called *Living with the Fog*.

Psychiatric symptoms

Personality changes

Another symptom not usually attributed to B_{12} deficiency affects the personality of the sufferer. This often manifests as **sudden mood swings**. Altogether, 58% of those who took part in the survey had experienced this and had displayed sudden changes in behaviour that caused all manner of problems, not just in the domestic setting but also in the workplace (more of this later). I'm not aware of any research that has been conducted into why people suddenly begin to behave unpredictably, but I do know that left untreated vitamin B_{12} deficiency does cause severe mental health problems, often leading to episodes of psychosis.[11]

Bethan's story

The telephone call that I took began all too familiarly. 'I'm 82 and have been having B_{12} injections every month for the past 38 years. I had major stomach surgery when I was in my mid-40s and the surgeon told me that I would need them for life. Now they've stopped them altogether.'

I asked Bethan why her GP surgery had suddenly stopped her life-giving treatment.

'Well, a new chap started and he told me that I couldn't possibly continue having monthly injections and that I would have to wait three months between having one. I created a bit of a fuss and he said that he would check my B_{12} levels and take it from there. Well, I went back to discuss my results, which I was sure would be low and he told me that I had far too much B_{12} in my blood and they couldn't possibly give me any more as it would be too dangerous. He said he would check my levels in three months' time. Three months later I went back for another blood test feeling dreadful, tired, unable to concentrate and generally groggy. This time my B_{12} levels had fallen but were still within what the guidelines stated. He said that I no longer needed the injections.'

There was little I could offer Bethan other than to suggest that she ask to see another GP or maybe consider taking B_{12} supplements in the form of sub-lingual methylcobalamin lozenges or sprays.

Six months later I had a call from Bethan's friend. 'Bethan's in hospital,' she said. 'She's been detained under section three of the Mental Health Act.'

Bethan's friend was her only friend. Bethan had no family and only saw her friend once a week when they both attended the local church. I was given the telephone number of the hospital where Bethan was being detained and later on in the day telephoned the ward and asked to speak to Bethan.

'Please help me,' she cried over the telephone. 'They still won't give me any B_{12} and I'm sure that is why I am here.'

I visited Bethan at the hospital in the West Country and took her Get

Well cards sent by concerned members of the Pernicious Anaemia Society along with some flowers to brighten the room that she was in. Two weeks later Bethan had an appeal against her detention. I attended it with Bethan and the solicitor who had been appointed to her. The appeal was held in a large room in the hospital. I learing it was a judge, a GP, a lay-person, the psychiatrist looking after her and a nurse. I informed the judge of the link between B_{12} and psychosis and he asked the psychiatrist why she hadn't been given any B_{12} if she had been receiving it for so many years. 'Her serum B_{12} is not below the threshold used to determine deficiency,' the doctor informed the judge who then asked me if it was possible to overdose on the vitamin. I told him that it was impossible and that celebrities regularly received intravenous infusions of B_{12}. We were asked to leave the room while the panel made their decision. During the break in proceedings I asked the psychiatrist if Bethan might have some methylcobalamin sub-lingual lozenges that I had brought with me. He took the lozenges, but told me that wasn't possible.

Bethan's appeal was turned down by the panel and it was good that it was so. Bethan was still suffering from delusions about her neighbours.

'But,' said the judge, 'we have decided to restart the B_{12} injections.' Bethan received two weeks of loading doses and at the end of the third week of treatment she was discharged. Her possessions now included the methyl-cobalamin sub-lingual tablets that I had asked her doctor to give her – they had not been given to her but were placed with her other possessions that had been removed from her. She is now on monthly injections again after I had written to the senior partner in the surgery that she is registered with. I also wrote to the head of psychiatric services in her area and received a reply thanking me for bringing this problem to his attention and that injections of B_{12} would be given every month for the rest of Bethan's life.

Bethan is still living at home and has not been re-admitted.

More usually, these personality changes lead to breakdown in relationships and marriage, usually because the sufferer's doctor will not associate the mood swings with the patient's pernicious anaemia. Consequently, and perhaps more importantly, the patient's family, friends and workplace colleagues will not realise that the personality changes are a consequence of him or her having pernicious anaemia either. This is despite reports of this in the scientific literature. To quote from a report published in 2003:

> Psychiatric manifestations are frequently associated with pernicious anaemia including depression, mania, psychosis, dementia.[12]

And often the psychiatric manifestations occur before pernicious anaemia has been diagnosed:

> Psychiatric manifestations can occur in the presence of low serum B_{12} levels but in the absence of the other well recognised neurological and haematological abnormalities of pernicious anaemia. Mental or psychological changes may precede haematological signs by months or years. They can be the initial symptoms or the only ones. Verbank et al described the case of a patient with vitamin B_{12} deficiency in whom hypomania, paranoia and depression had successively presented during a period of five years before anaemia had developed.[13]

The authors (Professor Dollfus's team at Caen University in France) conclude that all psychiatric patients should have their B_{12} status evaluated before any treatment begins:

> We recommend consideration of B_{12} deficiency and serum B_{12} determinations in all the patients with organic mental disorders, atypical psychiatric symptoms and fluctuation of symptomatology. B_{12} levels should be evaluated with treatment resistant depressive disorders, dementia, psychosis or risk factors for malnutrition.[14]

Nominal aphasia

'Nominal aphasia' describes the inability to recall the name of persons or things. This was reported by 49.8% of sufferers responding to the Society's survey. As with other symptoms, the severity will vary from person to person, with some sufferers experiencing problems in recalling names only now and again, whilst others struggle to remember the name of family and friends or what everyday objects are called.

Linked to this are general **confusion** and **poor concentration** (74.9%) along with **'handbag in the fridge'** syndrome, where the sufferer places objects in unusual places. **Memory loss** to a greater or lesser degree was reported by 78.4%. Less common, but linked to the above, 21.9% of respondents to the survey had experienced **suicidal thoughts**.

Heightened emotions

Also known as **'tear jags'**, the sufferer gets very emotional for little or no reason. Sometimes he or she will just find themselves crying for no reason. I'm unaware of any explanation for this, but perhaps it is because sufferers feel that their situation is so hopeless because, despite having injections to replace vitamin B_{12}, the symptoms don't go away either at all or completely.

Neurological symptoms

Left untreated, B_{12} deficiency can lead to serious and *irreversible* nerve damage to the peripheral nerves (the nerves in hands and feet – 'peripheral neuropathy') and eventually the central nervous system (the spinal cord). This is why it is so important that any symptoms should be investigated immediately and that the current tests used to determine B_{12} deficiency and pernicious anaemia should be thoroughly revised and updated. As I have said previously in 2013, the National External Quality

Assessment Service (NEQAS), the body that oversees the quality of laboratory testing in the UK, issued the following B_{12} 'alert':

False normal B_{12} results and the risk of neurological damage: *B_{12} assays may be vulnerable to interference resulting in normal values despite severe cobalamin deficiency. Where there is discordance between the clinical features of neuropathy – parasthesiae, loss of joint position sense, or megaloblastic anaemia and a 'normal' B_{12} result – clinicians are advised to request storage of serum for further testing and are advised to treat the patient with B_{12} replacement therapy. Further testing may include repeat testing by an alternative B_{12} assay, holotranscobalamin assay, serum methylmalonicacid and measurement of intrinsic factor antibody. Treatment with B_{12} should not be delayed to avoid progression of neurological damage…..*

In other words, if a patient has suspected nerve damage due to possible pernicious anaemia or low B_{12} levels yet the test shows a 'normal' B_{12} level, doctors are advised to ignore the test result and commence replacement-therapy with B_{12} injections in order to prevent any further neurological damage.

Pins and Needles (paraesthesia)

Tingling felt in the hands and feet can be the first sign of nerve damage due to B_{12} deficiency (reported by 65.7% of respondents), and can lead to numbness in any part of the sufferer's body, but is felt usually in the feet. Clumsiness (65.8%) often manifests itself in the patient continually bumping into walls, which Pernicious Anaemia Society members know as the 'shoulder bumps' (48.4%), while 59.5% had experienced **dizziness** and 33.2% suffered from **vertigo**. One of the most common problems that patients with nerve damage due to their pernicious anaemia will encounter is donning underwear or hosiery, because balance problems standing on one leg or bending down cause all manner of difficulties. This has become known among members of the Pernicious Anaemia Society as 'the knicker dance'. Another little-known consequence of B_{12} deficiency is a burning sensation in the legs and feet, known as 'Grierson-Gopalan syndrome'. This was reported by 33.4% of respondents

Conclusion

There are serious issues in establishing whether someone has vitamin B_{12} deficiency and whether the deficiency is due to pernicious anaemia. There is a need for the symptoms associated with B_{12} deficiency to be revised and disseminated to physicians so that they can identify it and actively look for signs of any deficiency. Failure to recognise any deficiency leads to misdiagnosis or patients being left without any explanation for their condition – sometimes for many years, during which time they are at risk of developing serious and irreversible nerve damage.

Chapter 3

Workplace issues for people with pernicious anaemia and vitamin B$_{12}$ deficiency

We have seen in the previous chapters that the symptoms of pernicious anaemia are varied and many. However, not only is there a wide range of symptoms, but also the *extent* to which any individual symptom is experienced varies, with some patients experiencing only a few of the symptoms, and experiencing them only slightly, whilst others can tick off the whole long list of symptoms and experience some or all of them intensely. If you like think of the symptoms as a row of cans in a supermarket, with each can at the front of the shelf being one of the wide range of symptoms, then think about how deep those rows of cans may reach back into the shelves – that is the equivalent of how intensely the symptoms can be experienced. Some of the cans go back just two cans deep while others are 20 deep. And, just as different sufferers experience a different variety of the symptoms and to different intensities, so will they experience different levels of problems in the workplace. Some people with pernicious anaemia will find allowances are made for their condition whilst others will struggle to carry on with their work. How people are affected will depend on how many of the symptoms they have and how intensely they experience them – it's all about the individual.

The extent to which pernicious anaemia affects the way in which patients carry out their job will also be affected by the type of work involved and whether it is compatible or incompatible with the symptoms experienced by the individual. So, a person who is still experiencing 'the sighs' and is not able to breathe properly will find that his or her manual job will be difficult, if not impossible, to carry out because any physical exertion causes problems. Meanwhile, those who rely on their mental capabilities to carry out their work will struggle, to some degree or other, to carry on with their career if they still experience 'the fogs'. Many people with pernicious anaemia will not have problems at work because their symptoms will have disappeared with the start of treatment. However, many, though nobody knows just how many, will still have some or all of their symptoms but will be able to carry on because the symptoms do not affect the tasks they have to do. Usually, 'the strange tiredness' will never fully disappear, and the sufferer will have days when the tiredness is not as bad as others, but it is the *degree* of tiredness that will determine how work is affected. This is what makes it so difficult to categorise the symptoms of pernicious anaemia and to produce a set of guidelines on how to manage the condition in a work situation – every patient is different to some degree.

The most problematic symptoms

There are three symptoms in particular that can have a serious impact on the sufferer's working environment and which I have repeatedly come across. The first of these concerns the sudden, unexpected **mood swings** that many patients experience. Erratic behaviour and sudden outbursts are bad enough at home, where family and friends might understand the patient's frustrations, but in the workplace they can cause all manner of problems. Colleagues can be left feeling hurt and confused, and the sufferer embarrassed and frustrated. Yet the sufferer's behaviour will not usually be attributed to his or her pernicious anaemia and can and does lead to disciplinary proceedings.

The second symptom is one that crops up repeatedly in letters in my in-tray at the Pernicious Anaemia Society – sudden, unexpected bouts of **diarrhoea**. This can mean that the employee has to leave meetings suddenly, becomes distracted in conversations, and unfortunately can lead to very embarrassing situations. It can also lead to anxiety about undertaking journeys away from the convenience of the workplace facilities, and this in itself causes more problems.

The third symptom that causes problems in the workplace is the desire and need for some patients to escape the hub-bub of everyday working life and seek solitude and peace and quiet. For some, getting away from the constant stream of information and questions can be easy, but for others it is impossible and not being able to cope with what soon becomes information overload, and the demands made by fellow workers, leads to more mood swings, impatience and irrational behaviour, as described above. Again, this is made worse by colleagues not fully understanding the true nature of pernicious anaemia and recognising that the sufferer will sometimes need to find somewhere away from the bustle of everyday life.

Any individual with pernicious anaemia who is still symptomatic even after treatment has started, will come up against one major hurdle when dealing with employers – they, the employers, won't be aware that pernicious anaemia causes any problems once it has been diagnosed and treatment started. And to make matters worse, the chances are that, if the problems end up being discussed at an employment tribunal, neither will the sufferer's trade union or other representatives.

So what can be done?

If you are struggling to continue in employment after treatment for vitamin B_{12} deficiency has begun, there are a number of options that can be explored. These may seem unrealistic in your situation, but it is important to consider all the possibilities that might just work.

Negotiate an employment schedule that works for you

The first of these is to try to negotiate with your employer for a work-scheme that takes into consideration your condition. Even though the current economic situation makes this difficult, it is not impossible to change the nature or hours of work so that the impact of your condition on work performance is minimised. That's what happened to me, though only for a year. When I was eventually diagnosed, I was able to negotiate with my employers (the college where I was a lecturer) to have all of my lectures in the mornings so I could go home to rest at around 1:30, with no evening class commitments. Sadly, that only lasted a year and when I was put back to a full-day timetable, with two post-graduate evening classes, I lasted just six weeks before collapsing.

There have been instances where employers have made amendments to the sufferer's working day and the mutually agreed arrangements have worked well. Again, it will all depend on the individual's symptoms, circumstances and the nature of the job.

Personal experiences

Just before writing this I checked the Pernicious Anaemia Facebook page where the day before I asked for examples of patients having workplace problems. Here's a small selection of the posts:

'I ended up having eight months off work before they diagnosed me.'

'I lost my job due to my PA. Have nerve damage and ongoing symptoms.'

'Have just left my job as a teacher. It's been impossible to work the 50+ hours a week needed to keep on top of things. In my last week I knocked coffee over onto my keyboard five times. I am forever walking into things, knocking things etc. The worst days are when the aphasia hits and I can't remember what everyday objects are called, though my class always thought that was pretty funny.'

'I'm off work three years.'

'I just resigned today.'

There are plenty more small snippets on the Society's Facebook page, but for more detailed accounts, read the postings on the online forum that can be found on the website.

Top tip

Go to www.pernicious-anaemia-society.org and click on the 'Information for Employers' tab. Download the information sheet and print it off, then go to the 'Symptoms checklist' under the Symptoms tab. Read through the symptoms and tick those that apply to you – you may be surprised at just how many you are experiencing. On a new sheet of paper list all those symptoms that you have ticked on the checklist. Make an appointment to discuss your symptoms with your employer, or with the Human Resources department, and take along to the meeting the

'Information for employers' leaflet plus your list of symptoms. Hopefully, this information will help your employer understand your medical condition and allow the negotiation of a working environment based on your individual needs and capabilities.

But what if your employer cannot, or will not, make any changes to your working environment? Well, there are a number of different avenues that can be explored.

Employment tribunals

As I have just mentioned, grievances by either the employer or employee sometimes end up being arbitrated at an employment tribunal or similar. If this happens, then the real battle will be to convince the panel that it is through no fault of your own that you are unable to continue to do what you were originally hired to do. This can be extremely difficult and frustrating if your employer calls in a doctor to give his or her opinion because, unless you are extremely fortunate in that doctor being a fellow sufferer, almost inevitably he or she will state that once replacement-therapy injections of B_{12} have been started, sufferers will no longer have the symptoms of pernicious anaemia and can live a normal life. To make matters worse, there are people who have pernicious anaemia and *do* manage to live a perfectly normal life after their injections have begun; they are able to say goodbye to all of their symptoms and will be sure this must be true for other sufferers. However, all is not lost. The Pernicious Anaemia Society provides a service to their members whereby the Chairman (that's me at the time of writing) writes a letter in support of the sufferer that can be presented to the tribunal. I've written around 20 of these in the last six months, which led to positive results in around 15. I cannot be specific, of course, but I can say that many people with vitamin B_{12} deficiency, contrary to what is normally believed. still remain symptomatic after treatment has begun. It can help in individual cases, but what really needs to happen is for society at large to become aware of this issue.

Assessment for work incapacity benefit

The UK's benefits system will undergo significant changes in the coming years and benefits claimants face the prospect of undergoing a thorough assessment as to their capability to work. The Pernicious Anaemia Society is able to help by providing an explanation of how the disease can lead to severe physical disability as well as reduced cognitive function. As with employment tribunals, this takes the form of a letter written by me. If you have developed any neurological damage due to being deficient in B$_{12}$ for a long period of time, whether due to misdiagnosis or not, then it becomes easier to convince any assessor of the need for assistance in getting around.

There are of course varying degrees to which any neurological damage will affect the mobility of any sufferer. More difficult is convincing the assessors that any cognitive issues that you have are attributable to pernicious anaemia, as cognitive impairment is not widely acknowledged as being caused by a paucity of B$_{12}$.

Jennifer's story

I was diagnosed with pernicious anaemia in November 2012. I was living in London until the end of February 2010. At that point I moved to South Africa to get out of the rat race. I was sick and tired of the Tube and had always been quite tired at the end of every day for a couple of years before that; I put it down to city living and working hard, but now I think it was the start of my illness. At one point sitting at my desk in London, probably around November 2009, tinnitus started in my left ear, simply out of nowhere and lasted for two hours. I even mentioned it to my boss. It went away and that was that.

I moved to South Africa on Saturday February 27 2010, and started work on the Monday. I was staying at my mother-in-law's house until my husband could join me and move into our own house. I was tired – weary – and going to bed quite early; I was always in bed by 9 pm but put it down to the fresh sea air as we now lived on the coast.

In July 2010, I began to have what I now know were gall bladder attacks and I had my gall bladder removed in September 2010. While I was recovering from the surgery, which was no issue, our stuff from London arrived and we finally moved into our house. It was a big house which needed a lot of work doing to it. Over the next 11 months I had the combined pressure of the house renovation, running a guest house, working full-time, a decrease in finances from London as we were establishing ourselves in a new place, living in a new country, cultural changes and moving from London to a small town. In addition, my husband's father fell terminally ill. I was exhausted to the point of going to bed very early most nights. My body was also learning to cope without my gall bladder and I had some digestion issues for approximately one year.

In March 2012, I noticed that I was not hearing clearly on my left side. As a young child I had had hearing problems and put it down to that. I went to see an ENT specialist, who advised me that my ears were fine and there was a problem in my head. He wanted to rule out a tumour as I did not have dizziness, which is usually associated with other hearing loss issues and I had a quick MRI. No tumour – he said. He thought maybe I had an inner ear virus and gave me Serc [a drug containing betahistine dihydrochloride] to increase blood flow to my inner ear as I had a 50% hearing loss.

About six days later, the dizziness hit with a vengeance. I would stand up and almost fall over. Then I started to drop things – a lot. Then I could not think of words. Who forgets the word for 'dog'? I did. I believe I referred to my dog as 'that furry thing on four legs that barks'. Then I thought, 'Hmmm..., I need another opinion'. I went to see an inner ear specialist who did some tests and diagnosed me as having shingles on my brain. Then he told me that it was a brain virus that would take up to six months to clear but my symptoms were those of shingles in my brain.

Well..., after six months things were worse. I was beyond tired. I had what the Pernicious Anaemia Society refers to as that 'strange tiredness'. I would fall into a dead sleep and wake up between 1 am and 5 am and be unable to sleep – then be exhausted for the day. This went on for months. I had headaches that lasted for days. My calf muscles hurt a lot. I was still dizzy but I think the Serc helped reduce the severity of that. Tons of vertigo though, and I could not look at motion. Everything was too much for me. I would look at a load of laundry and think, 'I can't do it.' When one runs a guest house, there is a lot of laundry, so it is necessary to keep up with it! At my full-time job, things had changed in terms of the company. The new company was dreadful, but I took it to the extreme. I hated it with a passion because of the way in which the new bosses came in. Anger was ripping into me every day I had to be there. I normally can handle most things, but I was in an internal rage so strong I could not handle it. I never fully emoted this professionally, but I certainly had a negative attitude towards the company whilst maintaining my professionalism. However, had I been well, I think I would have been less full of anger and done something about it.

I had periodic facial numbness on my left side.

My deafness came and went on my left side. I asked the ENT specialist I had seen if this was part of the brain virus. He said it was as the virus attacks cranial nerves. It was now at the seven-month point. I woke up early one morning and I was blind in my left eye. It lasted for approximately 15 minutes and then my sight was back. I went flying over to the optician who looked in my eye and said he could not see anything – my pressure was normal. I called the ear specialist again, who then referred me to a neurologist.

I finally got an appointment in October 2012 and he sent me for a battery of tests over the next eight weeks. He was very thorough. I saw an otolaryngologist who did three hours of tests on my vestibular system, I had a 90-minute MRI where they also shot dye into my veins to look at my brain vessels, and a cardiologist tested my heart and gave me a 'transoesophageal echocardiogram' in ICU. I spent the night in hospital for that one. I had a heart monitor, blood tests, and a lumbar puncture that showed my pressure to be 250 so it was thought I had hydrocephalus and needed a shunt.

When the blood test results came in for pernicious anaemia, I was at 109 for B_{12}. The doctor called me and said I had pernicious anaemia and that I would be on injections for the rest of my life. 'Go and get one right now, and then have one a month.' This was, remember, in South Africa. I began to do this, but got shots every week as there you can simply go to the pharmacy clinic and pay R30 for a shot when you want one (that is about £2). After about one month I started to feel something bubbling up inside me which I now think of as my life and energy coming back. Thankfully I regained the sight in my left eye.

I came to London six weeks later for a six-month month work contract, which was when I discovered the Pernicious Anaemia Society website. I joined and began to research this illness. Through the site, I learned about folate, which I had not been told to take by the doctor in South Africa. I began to take it and six weeks later, which is as I write, I feel like a million bucks! However, I still cannot handle looking at motion, even when feeling well.

Recently I noticed my eyesight had massively changed for the worse, as I get my optician to check my vision once per month, so we also have a record of this change. I went to an ophthalmologist who confirmed that my optic nerves in both eyes are pale and anaemic. He feels that folate will help as I have only just started to take it in the last month, but this is being monitored as my eyesight is not as good as it was.

I need shots much more frequently than every three months, but as I go home to South Africa once a month, I get a shot there and I also supplement with patches and take the Methyl B_{12} lozenges under my tongue. I still do get symptoms – as I approach the fourth week from my last shot, I begin to get dizzy and have tinnitus – but by then I know I will be back in South Africa shortly and can get the injection when I land.

It is thanks to the Pernicious Anaemia Society that I feel so well! The forums are great!

Radical change

What if an employment tribunal decides that you are able to carry out your duties and you are faced with struggling on with the threat of dismissal for underperformance ever present? Well, this is where you are forced to make serious and radical decisions about your future. There are a number of options available.

One possible option is to retrain and change career (easier said than done if you are still symptomatic) to one that offers a more flexible working environment. This isn't easy, especially if your symptoms sometimes last more than one day, but such jobs can be found. The downside is that these jobs are almost inevitably poorly paid and the work can be erratic.

Perhaps a more radical solution is to become self-employed. In an ideal situation you will then be able to tailor your work pattern around your symptoms. However, it is only theoretically true that you will be able to choose what hours to work; in practice, the times you work will be determined by when and how your symptoms manifest themselves. As I write this, it is approaching 11 o'clock in the morning and I know that I have around 30 minutes of writing time left before I start to type sentences that won't make sense when I read over them. That's why I write in the mornings and why I go to the Pernicious Anaemia Society's office in the morning. Around lunchtime I get very, and this is a strange way of putting it but it's the best I can do, I get very 'woozy'. It is my intention, when we – the Pernicious Anaemia Society – have succeeded in changing the way people regard pernicious anaemia, I am going to write highly erotic novels that will make me a fortune. I am aware, though, that I will have to write them in the mornings as that is when I am largely symptom-free. The same might apply to any sufferer considering self-employment – the working hours will be pre-determined by when the symptoms manifest themselves.

Jean's story

I have had to give up work because of pernicious anaemia. I was diagnosed six years ago. Looking back, with the benefit of the knowledge I now have of the condition, I now realise that I have probably had a B_{12} absorption problem of some sort all my life, as I have always tired easily.

Prior to my diagnosis, I had quite a responsible job as an area manager for a national charity. I began to feel very tired and forget to do things. I just couldn't get around to doing tasks and developed a 'mañana' attitude which resulted in my going to meetings woefully unprepared and forgetting to do things at the right times. Obviously, this impacted on my work and I was criticised and formally disciplined. I just could not understand what was going on as I had always had a reputation for being quite dynamic and proactive before. I accepted the criticism as it was totally justified. Eventually, I found myself going into the office and..., well..., just sitting there, messing about on the computer, as everything seemed to be so much of an effort. Eventually I resigned because I knew I was about to be sacked for incompetence. This damaged my professional reputation irrevocably.

I consulted my doctor who prescribed anti-depressants. I did not take them. I got a job as a warehouse assistant at a large mail order company. This had a big impact on my finances, but I wanted to get away from having to be responsible for anything important and, to be honest, the fact that I was being told what to do all day and didn't have to think for myself came as something of a relief. I managed for about a year, though by this time I was unable to do anything outside work except sleep. I became more and more unsociable, rarely going out or seeing friends. Inevitably, my organisational ability was spotted and, with some trepidation, I accepted a more responsible job, though still quite a low grade one. This job was a fairly physical one and I quickly found that I could not keep up with targets and was exhausted and tearfully upset at the end of every shift. I was also making basic errors with paperwork and simple calculations. The crunch came one evening, at the end of my shift, when

I was completing a report that required some figure-work that I would have expected to be able to do in my head in about three minutes. It took me at least half an hour and I realised that I was not retaining any of the information I was reading. (This can still be a problem sometimes.)

I took time off sick, convinced that I had a dementia-related condition, and went to the doctors, presenting myself in floods of tears. Blood tests showed I had a B$_{12}$ deficiency and I was started on the injections. Initially the improvement was dramatic, but as time went on, I had to fight for more frequent injections and finally managed to get them every eight weeks. The story from here will be familiar to you. I changed doctors after a house move and was put back on 12-weekly injections and had to go through the whole thing again, being told by my doctor that I only wanted them more often because, 'They give you a buzz and you've heard that people like Madonna have them before performances to perk them up!' Having to defend yourself when at your lowest ebb is not the pleasantest of experiences.

Eventually, though the mental problems, dizziness and pins and needles did recede, I gave up work as I could not cope with the sudden fatigue, which requires an instant response, in the form of a nap. It is not easy to do that at work. I asked for a transfer to another job but was told this was not possible. Ironically, I was told that I had had too much 'casual' time off to be considered for this! I had been taking about two days off every month, which I spent in bed!

I took proper sick leave at this point, and my employment was eventually terminated three years ago on medical grounds after having my mental health queried with my doctor as well as the usual verification of my condition. The pay-off I received was small and I am now dependent on my partner financially as the condition is not recognised for benefit purposes due to the fact that I do not have 'significant' spinal cord involvement.

I do work from home, but only when I am fit to do so. On the face of it, and by ATOS criteria, I am physically and mentally fit for work, but for maybe two hours per day on about three days a week, and I never know when those days or times will be. I can't think of an employer who would be happy to employ me on that basis, however capable I am. Self-employment is the only option, and I am now earning about 20% of my previous career salary.

The psychological impact of not being financially independent has also had an effect on me and I am now far less confident than I used to be. I do not like being the reason why we can no longer afford holidays or replace our old car. Being so tired all the time really sucks.

Struggling on

Finally, there are many thousands of people with pernicious anaemia in employment and following careers who have not made any significant changes to their working lives. This could be because they simply cannot, because no allowances or changes can be made and they can just about manage to hold on. It could be because they might not want to acknowledge that they are having problems and they keep struggling to carry out what is expected of them. I remember one of the first members to join the Society, who was a secondary school teacher, telling me that when she gets home after struggling to cope with the daily pressures of modern teaching, she opened her front door, locked it behind her, and headed straight for bed. That made me think just how many other sufferers must follow a similar lifestyle. I don't think we shall ever know.

Conclusion

If you are still experiencing the symptoms of pernicious anaemia, to whatever extent, then you will need to make some changes to the way in which you carry out your work. These changes can be small and easy to make, or you may face life-changing decisions that will affect your and your family's lives for many years to come. There is a serious lack of understanding among employers of how pernicious anaemia can still be a problem for employees even after B$_{12}$ replacement-therapy injections have commenced. People with pernicious anaemia who are still symptomatic will encounter problems not only in the workplace, but also, to some degree or other, in their home and family life. That is what we shall now examine.

Chapter 4

The impact of pernicious anaemia and vitamin B_{12} deficiency on family life

A few years ago I was wandering around a supermarket, pushing my trolley and minding my own business when I happened upon the parents of a friend from my schooldays. I was asked what I was doing these days and I quickly related my story of how I had had to give up my career and that I now ran a charity.

'Oh, what is the charity?' they asked.

'It's a patient support group for people with pernicious anaemia,' I replied, expecting to hear the usual 'Oh, my grandmother had that.' Instead they both looked astounded and said, 'Our Jane has that. She's in a terrible state. She's sleeping all the time, and because she keeps forgetting to pick the kids up from school there's the chance that they'll be taken into care.'

Now I had long been aware that people who are still symptomatic after starting B_{12} replacement injections often have problems at home. I had heard of many marriage breakdowns, other relationship breakdowns and all manner of trouble as one partner struggled with the worst aspects of the disease, but this was the first time that I realised the true extent to which families can be affected by the condition. I told my friend's parents to ask their daughter to contact me, which she did a few days later. I was able to give her the contact details of a doctor in the area who uses B_{12} infusions to treat still symptomatic patients. I am pleased to report that she made an almost miraculous recovery.

She is now back at work and picks up her children without any problems. I do not know what would have happened if I had not bumped into her parents that day at the supermarket, but I suspect the situation with the local social services would have deteriorated to some extent or other.

Just as we have seen that people who are still symptomatic after starting treatment often have problems in their workplace, they will also often encounter problems in their home life. Again, these problems will vary in intensity depending on just how severe the symptoms are. They can range from needing to take an afternoon nap to not being able to socialise in any form and experiencing a complete personality change – I have heard them all.

As with workplace issues, a big factor in domestic problems is the generally false assumption that B$_{12}$ injections will reverse all symptoms. Sufferers are told to expect this, and become frustrated and desperate if it does not happen. Their friends and families expect it, and have little patience when exhaustion, mood swings and mental fog do not go away. Being aware that for many sufferers symptoms remain, or require much more frequent B$_{12}$ treatment, can make a major difference to all the problems I am going to describe.

Domestic strife

If one of the partners in a marriage or relationship develops pernicious anaemia and he or she continues to be symptomatic despite standard treatment, this can cause friction in the relationship for one of several reasons. Just as sufferers in this position will have had to make changes to the way in which they work, they will also have to make changes to their home life. Again, the severity of the symptoms will determine the extent to which home life is affected. I will take a look at how the most common symptoms can mean that family life will no longer be the same as it used to be.

The strange tiredness

The most common change that is noted when a family member is still symptomatic after treatment has begun is an altered sleep pattern. This can manifest itself in various ways and can include the need to sleep during the day, going to bed very early or rising very late. One member of the Pernicious Anaemia Society coined the saying, '*The Archers* and bed', referring to the popular radio programme that airs for 15 minutes at 7 pm each weekday evening on BBC Radio 4. I go to bed before then so have to catch up with the goings on in Borchester by listening to the earlier edition broadcast at 2 pm.

This need for early nights or late mornings causes much embarrassment among some sufferers as they fear they might be regarded as lazy. This embarrassment disappears when they come together in a group; then individuals readily reveal how they manage the strange tiredness.

Obviously, the need for sufferers to go to bed very early will have an impact on their social lives, especially if the option of rising later in the morning is not available due to work or family commitments. And whilst the individual may prefer to take to his or her bed rather than attend some evening social event, his/her partner may not want to forgo the opportunity to socialise during the evening. This can and does lead to strains within many relationships.

One way around this is for the couple to base their social life around the patient's sleeping requirements and, for example, to make sure that any socialising is carried out during the daytime. This is how I cope. I don't have dinner dates but have lunchtime meetings; I go to the cinema (usually empty cinemas) during the daytime and visit other attractions when I am not feeling the worst effects of the strange tiredness. Again, these options are not available to all patients and their partners, which can lead to problems. Managing the strange tiredness becomes even more complicated when family get-togethers are involved. Whilst christenings or weddings are not usually a problem for the early-to-bed brigade, other family gatherings that take place in the evenings can and do prove to be a problem, not least because of the risk of appearing rude and offending family members who might interpret any non-attendance as a snub. There is a way around this but it is not an easy fix. You will have to educate family members about your condition – and that can take years. In the best cases, the fact that the sufferer is still symptomatic and behaves in a way that seems slightly odd is treated as a joke by other family members. It is better to be regarded as eccentric than to cause upsets within the family group. Another way to alleviate any possible bad consequences of not attending a family gathering is to try to visit those who are celebrating something in the evening, in the morning or afternoon instead; best wishes and presents can be given, and apologies for not attending the event in the evening, and consequently no offence will be taken. However, this problem of not being able to attend evening events will be more difficult for family members to understand if they know of another person who has pernicious anaemia who is completely non-symptomatic. If this is the case then you could do worse than show family members this book and hope they will then understand why you cannot attend in the evening. This issue is, however, further complicated when some patients are perfectly able to attend evening events but need to sleep in the afternoon. There is no one-size-fits-all in pernicious anaemia.

Sudden mood swings

Sudden mood swings are one of the most underrated symptoms of pernicious anaemia. Again, they affect people differently even after treatment to rectify the B$_{12}$ deficiency has commenced. The impact this will have on a relationship will, of course, depend on how understanding your partner and family are and whether they attribute these mood swings to your medical condition rather than to your erratic personality. To make family members aware of this behavioural symptom will again be a case of educating them by openly discussing this issue.

In the best case scenario, family members will make light of these sudden changes in personality. However, for some families the mood swings are so severe and the sufferer's behaviour so nasty that it can and does lead to relationships ending or the sufferer being isolated within the family group.

Loss of libido

It is only recently that loss of libido has come to light as an issue in B_{12} deficiency – but it now appears to be a common problem. I have not encountered any male members of the Pernicious Anaemia Society owning up to suffering from this; it appears to be an exclusively female problem, but this could be due to men being reluctant to discuss their health problems in general and their sexual health in particular.

Susan's story

Susan lived locally to me in South Wales and telephoned me to ask if she could have a word in private. I was completely unprepared for what she was about to discuss. She came into the Society's offices where I made her a mug of coffee. We went into my little private office and I closed the door. Her frankness surprised me.

'I have absolutely no libido and haven't for the past three years. My husband keeps threatening to leave me,' she told me, before asking, 'Is there anything I can do?'

I told Susan that I had never encountered this before and suggested that she talk to her doctor. It was then that I started to notice posts on the

Society's online forum about loss of sexual appetite due to the condition. I am guessing, but I think the main reason is because some patients never shake off the fatigue that they experience on a 24/7 basis.

Memory problems and 'nominal aphasia'

Problems with memory in general, and with forgetting the names for objects and of people, are both cognitive issues that may continue after treatment for B_{12} deficiency has started. While these can be troublesome in the workplace (see chapter 3), they do not usually cause problems in a family setting as mostly the family members will make light of your/the sufferer's inability to remember things or to recall what certain things are called. Yet again, it will all depend on the severity of these issues and the patience of the family members affected.

Desire for isolation, peace and calm

Many people who are receiving B_{12} replacement injections continue to want to be left in peace and to avoid any stress. Obviously this can cause ill feeling and give the impression the sufferer is an unfriendly, unsociable loner. At best such behaviour will be regarded as eccentric unless the family can understand that this is a result of vitamin B_{12} deficiency.

Sudden unaccountable bouts of diarrhoea

Many of the Society's members mention irregular bouts of violent diarrhoea as a particularly disabling symptom. Any time away from home needs to be planned carefully if the sufferer is likely to experience the sudden need to find a toilet. This is especially true on long car journeys and similar excursions. Although this problem will have an impact on the way in which the family operates, it is not usually a serious issue for the family members to accommodate and they are usually sympathetic to the needs of the sufferer and will gladly make the necessary allowances.

Housing issues

If the pernicious anaemia sufferer finds him or herself having to make a career change to a less strenuous job, or maybe even having to stop work altogether, then obviously the family finances will be affected to some degree or other. One of the saddest consequences of this will be that the family will have to make alterations to their lives, including in some cases moving into a smaller family home or into social housing. I know that many patients have had to move into accommodation that is more suited to their reduced income, but I suspect that many more are struggling to keep their current job just so that they keep the family home. I also know of several cases where sufferers who are single have had to move back home to live with their parents simply because they have had to give up work altogether.

Julie's story

At 10 years of age I became fatigued and detached and after numerous tests it was put down to a virus. I spent most of my time resting and missed a lot of school. At one point I was started on anti-seizure medication only to find out after an EEG that I was not epileptic. We named these episodes 'funny turns' as I could not explain how I felt. After two years I became stronger as the days went by and apart from fatigue and 'funny turns' every now and then I was almost back to feeling like me.

Pregnant at 18, I had a threatened miscarriage and could barely lift my head due to severe sickness; it was then that I stopped working.

I was referred to a specialist due to having a low BMI that I had had for numerous years, but nothing was detected. Everything went well throughout the pregnancy apart from an iron deficiency.

I had decided on a homebirth and was only allowed gas and air for pain relief, but it made me immediately feel unwell so I refused to take any more. From the moment I gave birth I became extraordinarily tired and struggled with night feeds. I would spend most of the day and night in bed and my husband and I decided I should stop breastfeeding.

Some months after giving birth I began to feel as though I had 'flu and the fatigue was like nothing I had experienced before. I felt faint, dizzy and sick. Doctors ordered some blood tests, assuming it was thyroid, but all tests came back normal and the cause was put down as viral.

After a few months, and lots of appointments later, the doctors diagnosed postnatal depression and I was started on an SSRI [a type of anti-depressant]; that night I had a severe reaction and I believed I was dying. I got through the night by taking some sleeping tablets and the next day the doctor started me on another anti-depressant. This anti-depressant helped me forget things for a while and I slept most of the time. When I became more aware again and my symptoms got worse, the doctor just increased the dose until I was on the highest possible.

Now I was passing out a lot and feeling so weak. I would wake in the night just shaking so much and my heart was beating so fast that if I dared stand I would faint. I was in and out of A&E. Sometimes it was blamed on low blood pressure, but many times on panic attacks. A full list of my symptoms included:

Fatigue

Palpitations

Tachycardia

Acid problems

Right-side weakness (comes and goes)

Vibration feeling through legs

Twitches throughout body

Sudden jerks of movement

Tingling and numb tongue and lips

Hand tremors

Muddling up words

Confusion

Swollen lymph nodes

Aches and pains

Sensitivity to food, light, noise, medication

Flushes

Fainting

This is not all of them, but all I can remember right now.

Many family members would tell me to 'snap out of it' as my child needed me and they believed I was a hypochondriac. I would phone my mum many times, crying for help, but she would tell me it was postnatal depression and it would get better.

After some months I was referred to a counsellor as my social life was affected by all my symptoms; after no improvement I was sent to a psychiatrist. I had one session with the psychiatrist who believed my problems were hormonal and suggested I try for another baby. I was now on sleeping tablets, diazepam and the highest dose anti-depressant and things still continued to get worse.

I decided it was time to stop all the medication as it certainly wasn't helping and I eventually gained the courage to speak to the practice manager, but all that came from that was a sick note signing me off for stress.

I began to see different doctors in the surgery, hoping one might find something, but I had a label now and it felt like no one wanted to help. One occasion when I went to the out-of-hours doctor, I was referred to a gastroenterologist to investigate my sickness and stomach pain. I never got a diagnosis, but they started me on omeprazole and domperodone. On another occasion in A&E they kept me in on an overnight monitor as my heart was fast and it still didn't go down when I was sleeping. They also found high liver enzymes. They wrote to the gastroenterologist and

I was dismissed. Upon checking my liver again it was normal and as a precaution I was sent for a 48-hour Holter monitoring test. The results showed slight tachycardia and many missed beats and I was referred to a cardiologist. The cardiologist gave me a heart scan and it came back normal; I was told it was due to anxiety and he said I was focusing too much on my health.

One night I woke with right-sided weakness and facial numbness. I was taken to A&E. They asked me about my symptoms and I explained about the severe weight loss. They did a few tests and all they found were ketones in my urine. I was discharged from hospital after no sleep at 7:30 am and with no bus fare. I had to ask someone for directions to the train station where my sister met me and drove me home.

A few months later I found out I was eight weeks pregnant but sadly miscarried. My GP suggested I try again, sooner rather than later. That also ended in miscarriage. They said it was common and I was otherwise healthy so refused to investigate why unless I miscarried again. It was then I decided to change GPs.

My new GP ordered many tests and put in a referral to a neurologist and endocrinologist. She actually believed me, but by this time my health was becoming worse and many days went by when I struggled to lift my head until I drank some sports drink. Given this impossible situation, my husband and I decided to move next door to his mother so we could get the help we needed.

After months of waiting for my appointments with the specialists I went to visit a new GP in the area I had moved to and found they had written to my old address. This meant I had to be referred again. The new referral was down as routine so I was told it would be a long wait. It was then my husband and I decided to try for another baby. Maybe the psychiatrist was right. I fell pregnant that month and I felt different this time and I had a strong feeling this one would not end in a miscarriage.

The fatigue was overwhelming; I fell to the floor in tears not knowing when I would be able to stand and feeling like I could not carry on. My husband phoned the doctors, who assured us it was perfectly normal.

I don't know how I got through those first weeks, but I did and I grew stronger. I started to feel normal and I was the healthiest I have ever been. My three-year-old daughter said, 'Mum, it is so nice to see you smiling.' She knew me as the mum who was always sleeping.

I saw the endocrinologist but as I was better I was dismissed. He told me to stay pregnant if it made me feel so good. I was very concerned that after the birth my symptoms would return.

As my pregnancy progressed I developed SPD [symphysis pubis dysfunction, causing pelvic pain] and my iron became low again. At seven months' pregnant I started to feel my heart go funny again, the worst it had ever been, and I started feeling detached. I ignored it as I believed if the doctors put it down to mental illness they might take my newborn child into care. I carried on and it was hard.

I saw the neurologist and he did a few tests and said he believed I was too young to have anything wrong. He advised that I should stop having children as they caused migraines, which can cause weakness. I was dismissed.

During a follow-up blood test my ferritin levels had risen but the doctors found macrocytosis. After reassuring the GP I did not drink alcohol they tested my B_{12}. It was below 50. I was finally started on cyanocobalamin, one daily.

At nearly nine months pregnant I was finding it hard to cope with my SPD and I was feeling really unwell. My midwife decided I should go to the hospital. I was given strong painkillers for the SPD and had a mental health assessment. It was decided I should be induced as they believed giving birth would stop me being anxious. I did not get a break from contractions and I had never felt pain like it. No anaesthetist was available and I had no choice but to take gas and air. The midwife told me my baby was back to back and that was causing the excruciating pain. I gave up on the gas and air as I felt too ill.

I finally gave birth in the early hours of the morning, but I felt so ill. My heart was so fast and missing beats. I tried to stand but fell back into a wheelchair that was near. The next day I still could not stand without the overwhelming feeling of dizziness and weakness. The midwives believed I was depressed. They gave me my own room and took some bloods. They all come back normal. I had no appetite and did not want any visitors.

The next day I went home and I was able to stand for a little longer. My symptoms got worse. I could not sit down for two minutes without my limbs falling asleep. I had vibrations through my legs most of the time and my short-term memory was non-existent. I didn't understand where I was, I was so confused. My lips and tongue were constantly numb now and my hair was falling out. Not only did I feel physically numb but also mentally numb. I felt like I couldn't carry on and the only way to prevent myself committing suicide was to stay in bed, telling myself that no matter how I felt I could not leave my girls without a mother.

A few weeks later a letter arrived asking me to go for an MRI. It gave me hope, but again nothing was found. I gave up breastfeeding so I could start on an SSRI, but after a few days I ended up in A&E; it was put down to anxiety but I believed it was the SSRI.

I went back to the GP complaining of symptoms, but was taken off the cyanocobalamin as my deficiency was believed to be pregnancy-related. I asked for further testing but it was refused. No follow-up needed, I was told. I was assigned a CPN [community psychiatric nurse] and I was then put on anti-psychotics, anti-depressants and diazepam.

I was at the doctors almost daily yet again, A&E and the out-of-hours. Eventually, after five months my B₁₂ was tested and it came back low. I was told to have a follow-up test in a month's time as just having one test is not reliable. I saw another GP in the practice and persuaded her to start me on injections.

I had my six loading doses. I felt no benefit to begin with but after six or seven weeks I started improving and eventually I felt like me again. I started to decline again when I needed an injection, so the GP referred me to an endocrinologist who said they did not specialise in pernicious anaemia and therefore could not authorise more injections. My GP now allows me to have an injection every 10 weeks. Now, seven months after my loading doses, most of my symptoms are back on a daily basis and one injection every 10 weeks is making no difference. My symptoms are certainly nowhere near as severe as before but they are difficult to live with. I have asked to be referred to a haematologist but my GP is seeking advice from my endocrinologist. My white blood count is low but it returned to normal after my loading doses. Since they have worn off it is low again, but comes back up to near normal after my injection. On my last blood test it showed neutropenia, but doctors put that down as viral. Looking back at all the blood tests, I have had a low white blood cell count all along.

Since becoming aware of B_{12} deficiency symptoms I have noticed some symptoms in my eldest daughter. The GP didn't feel it necessary to test her B_{12} level but we insisted. It came back just above 200. It is in the normal range and the GPs believe even my B_{12} being as low as 50 could not cause symptoms. When I visit my GP for anything now they say I am having a panic attack. My diagnosis has not changed a thing. I am concerned about both my daughters as I breast-fed my youngest with such a low level of B_{12} and I had just had nitrous oxide which depletes B_{12}.

I am hopeful the future will bring frequent injections according to the needs of each individual and better understanding and diagnosis for all struggling with B_{12} deficiency.

Conclusion

We have seen in this chapter how family life can be affected by symptomatic patients who have pernicious anaemia. The impact of the symptoms on family life will, of course, depend on their severity. In the worst cases, sufferers will encounter marriage break-ups and will feel even more isolated and frustrated at the lack of understanding of pernicious anaemia. In the best cases, the family will understand the nature of the disease and will make allowances for the sufferer so that he or she can lead as happy a life as is possible. But there are some family members who will have their own set of problems – children who have pernicious anaemia.

Chapter 5

Pernicious anaemia and vitamin B$_{12}$ deficiency in children and young people

Every day I come across stories of patients being misdiagnosed for many years before getting a correct diagnosis and starting treatment. I deal with the fallout of this problem on a daily basis in emails, telephone calls and posts on the Pernicious Anaemia Society's website, and on its Facebook pages. I have become used to the sad tales of suffering and how this has led to job losses, the ending of careers, and marriage and relationship break-ups. Stories that used to shock me no longer do so and are treated with a sense of resignation. After 10 years of listening to these problems I have, to some extent, become 'case hardened'. I have devoted myself tiredly rather than tirelessly to getting these issues resolved, but am well aware that whilst the Society has made enormous gains there is still a long way to go before the issues surrounding diagnosis and treatment are resolved.

There is, however, a group of patients whose stories and experience still move me to the point that I become angry – angry because, despite my almost constant efforts to get professionals to review how B$_{12}$ deficiency is diagnosed and treated, progress is far too slow. The group of patients that I am referring to are young people who have pernicious anaemia or are deficient in B$_{12}$ for some other reason. These sufferers are usually not in a position to stand up for themselves and have to rely on others to pass judgement on how they *should* feel and how they *will* be treated, with no options available to them. Unlike adults who need more frequent treatment regimes, young people will usually not be able to source alternative replacement-therapy, such as intravenous infusions, nasal sprays, sub-lingual drops or sprays, or pay for more frequent injections. And if they are still symptomatic after treatment to correct their deficiency has begun, they will often fail to enjoy their childhood and adolescence because they will be different from other young people; they may need to sleep more, find it difficult to concentrate and generally lack the energy that their peers will have in buckets. Furthermore, because their parents believe the family doctor who insists that once treatment has commenced their child will be quite capable of living a normal life, they will often have nobody to sympathise with them. This leads them to feel uncared for and unloved. Often, they will be labelled as having 'behavioural problems' because they don't want to participate in usual school-time activities and are unresponsive in the classroom during the afternoons when they start to experience extreme fatigue. These stories trouble me and frustrate me – as they do other sufferers who become aware of them.

Problems with diagnosis in young people

Just like other groups of people with pernicious anaemia, diagnosis is often a long time coming, and this delay is an even bigger problem in young people than it is in adults. This is because whilst doctors don't routinely actively look for pernicious anaemia as a possible cause of an adult's symptoms, they are even less likely to consider it in young person. This is because it is not as common in children and adolescents as in adults.

As with adults, the extent to which a child or adolescent will still experience the symptoms of B_{12} deficiency even after their treatment has begun will differ from individual to individual. Some will feel a little more tired in the days leading up to their injection whilst others will struggle to cope with everyday life on a daily basis. Some will enjoy their childhood and teenage years; others will have a daily battle with everyday tasks, finding refuge only when they take to their bed.

I have come to hear of the problems that children have from a variety of sources, but with children under the age of 11 it is usually from the mother, whilst I usually get to know of problems with teenagers up to the age of 18 almost exclusively from a concerned grandparent. Young adults over the age of 18 and under 23 usually contact me or other members of the Pernicious Anaemia Society themselves. I will deal with each of these groups in turn, but will first take a look at where it all begins – family planning.

Family planning

I am aware that people who have pernicious anaemia take their medical condition, and the genetic implications of it, into consideration when planning a family. Over the past five years I have known of a dozen or so members of the Pernicious Anaemia Society who have chosen not to have children because they do not want to take the risk of their child developing pernicious anaemia even if they were born fit and healthy. All of these cases involve women – I have yet to meet a man who has decided not to become a parent because of his disease. The exact genetic predisposition for offspring to inherit their parent's pernicious anaemia hasn't been fully explored or explained, with most of the research being rather vague but showing a familial link. Any decision on planning a family should therefore be made after an informed discussion has taken place between the prospective parents, perhaps taking into account any advice from medical professionals.

Newborns to 11 years

Whether a child is tested for B_{12} deficiency at birth will depend on where you live. In Canada's British Columbia, Alberta, Saskatchewan and Ontario, all newborns are tested to check the baby's B_{12} status, while in Quebec they use the urinary methylmalonic acid test (see page 12) to determine whether the baby is deficient in B_{12}. Babies in most of Europe aren't tested for B_{12} deficiency. In the UK, all parents are offered the heel prick test at birth, where blood is taken from the baby's heel and then screened to check for congenital hypothyroidism (CHT), cystic fibrosis (CF), medium-chain acyl-CoA dehydrogenase deficiency (MCADD), phenylketonuria (PKU) and sickle cell disorders (SCD). But not vitamin B_{12} deficiency.

Pernicious anaemia runs in families. Doctors have known this for decades and recent research has found that the brother or sister of a patient with pernicious anaemia is 40 times more likely to develop the disease.[15] It stands to reason therefore that patients who have pernicious anaemia will run the risk of passing on the condition to their children. Despite this, I am unaware of any routine test being carried out on the newborn babies of patients with pernicious anaemia. There's probably a good reason for not doing a blood test – the mother will have elevated serum B_{12} levels because she is receiving replacement B_{12} injections and this will distort any tests of the newborn's blood. In the Canadian provinces I mentioned above, they screen newborn babies for other indicators of B_{12} deficiency, but not serum levels. I am unaware of any plans to introduce regular screening of newborns for B_{12} deficiency in the UK.

Dorota's story

I received a telephone call in October 2012. It was from a young mother who, because of her accent, I believed was from Eastern Europe. 'I have pernicious anaemia,' she told me in a desperate voice, before adding, 'and my baby does too.' I offered the usual sympathies and then she told me the real reason for her call.

'I have a problem – I need more injections than every 12 weeks.' I told her that this was a very common problem and suggested that she ask her doctor for a 'therapeutic trial' of more frequent injections.

'Yes, yes, yes,' she told me in her broken English, 'he gives me injection ever six weeks.' I think I congratulated her but her story was only half finished.

'It's my baby,' she went on. 'He is going back to like he was before they discovered he had low B_{12}. He won't eat and he won't hold his head up, but they won't give him more injections until he goes low again.' The desperation that she was feeling could be heard in her voice. I simply didn't know what to suggest. The telephone went dead and I haven't heard from her since.

11 to 18 years old

The saddest cases I have had to deal with involve young people between the ages of 11 and 18 – those years when people leave their childhood behind and enter adulthood. It is a time of physical and mental change accompanied by ever-increasing responsibilities, expectations, commitments and freedom. Most people look back at their teenage years and remember a time of unbound energy and happiness, but for some adolescents who have pernicious anaemia it is a time of conflict, frustration and confusion. And their problems begin at the home:[vi]

vi Oddly enough it is grandmothers who tend to be the family member who contacts the Pernicious Anaemia Society and not the teenagers' parents. I offer no explanation for this.

Tom's story

Tom was an 11-year-old boy who had been diagnosed the year before his grandmother contacted us. Unusually there was no history of pernicious anaemia in his family. His parents had been told that it was unusual for pernicious anaemia to be found in young people but now that he was having an injection every three months everything would be fine.

'I notice him going downhill after about a month,' his grandmother told me on the 'phone. 'And in the weeks before his injection, his personality changes.' It was an all too familiar tale in adults and I couldn't see why this problem shouldn't manifest itself in young people too. I asked how Tom's personality changed in the weeks immediately before his injection.

'He becomes moody and angry with himself, and others,' she explained. 'And sometimes he just refuses to get out of bed. His behaviour in school also changes – and the teachers say that he becomes isolated and withdrawn and refuses to cooperate in the classroom.'

She went on to tell me that he was being referred to an educational psychologist and she feared he would be labelled as having behavioural problems. I wrote an explanatory letter to the head teacher of the boy's school stating that there were obviously problems with the current treatment regime. I don't know what happened after that, but I suspect Tom was labelled as having 'behavioural problems' – which might, of course, be the correct explanation for his behaviour. My concern remains that his erratic behaviour was caused by inadequate treatment and no amount of psychological support could replace the supplementary B₁₂ Tom might need.

Psychiatric problems and young people

Young people are also susceptible to psychiatric problems if they become deficient in vitamin B₁₂. Here's a letter written to the Canadian Medical Association in January 1976:

Chapter 5

Vitamin B$_{12}$ in late-onset psychosis of childhood

To the editor: I have recently found vitamin B$_{12}$ to be effective in treating children with late-onset psychosis. An 11-year-old girl, referred because of inability to get along with her peers, which had led to expulsion from a Girl Guides camp, showed typical features of late onset psychosis.[vii] *She had heard voices calling her name in the basement of her home and had attributed them to 'somebody playing tricks' on her. She claimed that other children were preparing to attack her and saying 'bad things' behind her back. On passing a total stranger in the street she asserted that she knew from his facial expression that he hated her. At home she was irritable, moody and uncooperative.*

She read the same fairy stories repeatedly and her drawing of a human figure was that of a queen in crown and robes. Her academic record was excellent and her intelligence quotient was 145 on the Peabody Picture Vocabulary Test.

Because she refused to take any medication apart from vitamins, I prescribed vitamin B$_{12}$ in an easily ingested form, not expecting that it would influence the psychosis. The plan was to substitute trifluoperazine when the habit of taking drugs twice daily had been established. On follow-up, after she had taken crystalline vitamin B$_{12}$ (Redisol), 75 g bid [twice daily] for 4 weeks, the delusions and hallucinations had ceased. Her mother described the results of treatment as 'amazing' and said, 'It's like having a different child in the house. I used to dread her coming in but now it's a happy home.'

This striking improvement has been maintained for more than 12 months and vitamin B$_{12}$, 75 to 125 µg bid, is the only medication

vii 1. Kolvin I: Studies in the childhood psychoses – diagnostic criteria and classifications. *Canadian Medical Association Journal* 1976; 114: 113.

that has been administered. When the drug has been discontinued or the dosage much reduced, the parents have observed that the patient becomes moody and irritable within a few days. Patients with late-onset psychosis usually respond to long-term treatment with phenothiazines, but since vitamin B_{12} produces no side effects or toxic reactions a trial of this drug for 2 or 3 weeks is recommended. Recent experience with other patients suggests that a combination of vitamin B_{12} and trifluoperazine is effective when there is an unsatisfactory response to the vitamin alone.

R. Denson, MSc, MD, CM, FRCP[C][16]

Domestic issues and juvenile pernicious anaemia

Teenagers with pernicious anaemia will face problems at home if they are still symptomatic after being diagnosed if family members are not aware that receiving treatment doesn't mean that the symptoms of the deficiency will necessarily disappear. As with adults, this issue is complicated by the fact that many young people who have juvenile pernicious anaemia *will* see their symptoms ease or vanish altogether, and this can further be complicated if the family's doctor reiterates and reinforces the common belief that the treatment to rectify the B_{12} deficiency will banish all the symptoms. Family members will often, though not always, believe the doctor.

So what happens then? Well, if the young person is still feeling the worst of the symptoms of pernicious anaemia – the extreme tiredness, cognitive impairment and sudden mood swings along with sudden severe bouts of diarrhoea – he or she will sleep a great deal more than his or her peers, won't want to socialise (because he or she won't be able to) and often he or she will be labelled (unfairly) as lazy. Then these still symptomatic young people will start having problems in school.

Issues with education

Just as adult patients with pernicious anaemia will encounter problems in the workplace but to varying degrees, so teenagers find themselves struggling with their education. Again, the extent to which the still symptomatic adolescent will encounter problems will depend on the severity and type of his or her symptoms. Most of the stories that I have heard revolve around the issue of the frequency of injections with the young person beginning to re-experience the symptoms of pernicious anaemia in the run-up to his or her next injection date. When the parent or grandparent suggests to the family doctor letting his/her child or grandchild receive the next injection sooner than the routinely prescribed three months, in all but a few cases the doctor will refuse. And any test conducted to determine the young person's B_{12} status will probably show healthy levels, which would seem to vindicate the doctor's decision not to sanction more frequent injections, just as he or she would do if adults requested more injections for themselves. However, whereas an adult can walk out of the doctor's surgery and find alternative sources of B_{12} (whether injections or not) and self-supplement, this option is not usually available to children – which means that they often endure the worst effects of pernicious anaemia more than their adult fellow-sufferers. Often, as the young person struggles in the weeks or days before the next injection is due, he or she will find it difficult to get up in the mornings. This leads to conflict with parents who trust the opinion of the family doctor and refuse to believe that their son or daughter could be suffering from the symptoms of pernicious anaemia as they have been told he or she is receiving adequate treatment to correct the deficiency in B_{12} that was the root cause of illness.

A further problem faced by many patients who have pernicious anaemia is getting through the day. A great many still symptomatic patients find it particularly difficult to cope with afternoons. I hear of adults who make it through their working day until around 1 pm but then simply stare at their computer screens until the end of the working day, hoping that nothing taxing will be asked of them. Other adults find that they need to sleep in the afternoons, some for many hours. Neither of these options will be available to schoolchildren who struggle in the afternoons. Instead they will often refuse to participate in school activities, won't be able to concentrate on their work and they are usually labelled as having 'behavioural problems'. This is especially true if the adolescent experiences sudden mood swings. Sometimes educational psychologists become involved. Obviously all of this will then have an impact on educational attainment, something that John experienced:

John's story, told by his family

John is a 12-year-old boy from Yorkshire. In July 2012 he badly broke his wrist and had nitrous oxide ('laughing gas') twice. During the six-week-long school holiday we started to see lots of changes in John. He didn't want to socialise with friends or family, and wouldn't meet up with friends. We originally thought this was because he was embarrassed at having a plaster cast on his wrist. He began to be withdrawn. He was really tired but struggled to sleep and woke during the night and early in the morning. Then there was the problem with his stomach – he started to experience very bad flatulence and episodes of repeated belching. Periods of constipation would be followed by episodes of diarrhoea.

In the September of 2012 he started secondary school and got more and more angry with us and himself. One minute he would be okay, then the next he would fly into a rage which could last quite a while. Then he started to forget things, and to forget what we had told him; he found it difficult to follow instructions and this is when his school work became affected as he was forgetting to do work or forgetting what he was told to do!

By the end of September I took him to the doctor, who wanted to refer him for his anger issues. He had blood taken. The results of the blood test showed that he had low white cells but they didn't know why. Earlier on in the year I had been diagnosed as having low B_{12} and so I asked for a copy of John's blood test results. The test showed that his haemoglobin was just above the low threshold and he also had low red blood cells.

I started to research more into B_{12} as I felt so ill myself. It was then that I started to see more and more of my symptoms in John. I became more convinced that John's problems were due to low B_{12}, but his doctor refused to take more blood because he was being referred to a consult-ant paediatrician. Then John started to develop more symptoms. His eyes began to hurt and he developed black bags under both his eyes. He experienced severe diarrhoea to the point that he was pooing himself – he hated going to school in case this happened. He began to experience tingling in his legs and he would spend days alone in his room refusing to socialise. It was hard for him to undertake any exercise as he became severely short of breath and would perspire excessively. And because he became worn out so quickly he didn't want to do anything.

This was now really impacting on his school work. He was forgetting books and couldn't revise for tests as his memory was so bad. This was awful because he had always been an A student. He couldn't do any out of school activities as he was constantly so tired and had no energy.

In December of 2012 he was seen by a consultant paediatrician, who was pleased to help us with his sleeping problems but was dismissive of my suggestion that his problems might be due to inadequate B_{12}. I had taken literature about B_{12} to the appointment, but the consultant wouldn't take it. John was prescribed 4 mg of circadin a night to treat his insomnia. The consultant eventually agreed to do more blood tests after much cajoling. John's red blood cells and white blood cells were now in range (only because his reference ranges had been changed because he had now turned 12 but they were still as low as previous results!) However, his B_{12} was 246 (the range is 211 – 911), while his folate was 5.9 (range 5.4 – 24). His haemoglobin was now low. I spoke to the consultant about his B_{12} and folate being low and just in range but he refused to treat him as he said he sees a lot of children who are iron-deficient at this age.

The tablets for insomnia worked, but his sleep was restless and he would always wake up early. I went to John's GP with my concerns about his low B_{12}, but was told they couldn't treat him because he was within the reference range – just.

I did more researching as I could see my son slipping away from us. He had changed from a loving confident boy to someone who we didn't recognise. I started arguing with my partner because he thought that John's behaviour was due to him attention seeking and just being naughty.

Eventually I went to my own GP with the suggestion that we have John take the 'Active' B_{12} test. He said he wanted to help as much as he could and he took the literature that I had brought to the appointment. He agreed to the B_{12} test being done as long as the local hospital could spin the blood. However, we would have to wait until after Christmas.

In January John had more blood taken. This was sent to St Thomas's for the active B_{12} test. The result showed his active B_{12} was low but within range and I was asked if they could measure John's methylmalonic acid (MMA). I agreed to this, but requested that if the MMA test didn't prove B_{12} deficiency, then John's homocysteine levels should be tested. This was agreed too. I heard nothing for over a week and thought that his MMA test must have proved that he was B_{12} deficient.[viii]

On 22nd January 2013 I received a call from our GP and was told that John was not deficient as his MMA was just in range at 275 (0–280) and his active B_{12} was 39; the lower threshold was 25.

I received a copy of John's blood results and phoned the helpline

---

viii Homocysteine is an amino acid. Amino acids are the building blocks of proteins and play a critical part in biological processes and nerve transmissions. A high level of homocysteine in blood is now considered a risk factor for heart disease, although there is still some debate as to how much of a risk this is. Low levels of B_{12} also lead to increased levels of homocysteine and there is a lively debate taking place as to whether levels of homocysteine should be used to determine B_{12} status rather than the currently used serum B_{12} test.

number on the report. I told a very helpful lady John's story and asked if the reference ranges were the same for children as they were for adults. She told me that at the moment they were, but should probably lower the MMA range (to 0–222) which would make John deficient. She said that she thought his B_{12} was very low for a boy his age as they had only changed the range for deficiency from 35 to 25 a few months previously which meant that if John's blood had been examined a few months before he would have only just been over the threshold for deficiency. We told her that we were cross that no homocysteine test had been done and nobody had phoned us. The lady agreed to phone our GP and class John as being sub-optimal as he couldn't be classed as fully deficient given he was just within the reference range for MMA until it could be changed for children.

That was when we had our first success. We saw John's GP who had read the literature I had taken him and was willing to trial him on cyanocobalamin tablets for one month. After that he agreed to test his blood and if he was under 800, then he would prescribe injections. He also agreed to prescribe iron tablets and folic acid tablets after I had explained to him that these needed to be at an optimum level for B_{12} to work. I asked him also to conduct the homocysteine blood test, but he couldn't understand what this would prove! I tried to explain but with no success.

We now informed John's school of his condition and gave them the Pernicious Anaemia Society literature along with other leaflets.[ix] I also provided them with the Society's symptoms list, with all his symptoms ticked, along with polyglandular literature and advised them to watch the You Tube video of diagnosing and treating B_{12} deficiency. They watched the video and couldn't believe a vitamin deficiency could be the cause of all of John's problems. John was now given a toilet pass to show in lessons and all teachers were informed of his needs.

---

ix The Society produces leaflets on Juvenile Pernicious Anaemia – one written for parents and one written for young people.

On 30th January we saw the paediatric consultant. He wasn't prepared to treat John's low B$_{12}$ as it was not his remit. As with other doctors, I presented him with some literature and again he wouldn't read it. He prescribed Movicol for John's constipation as he was still alternating between being constipated and having severe episodes of diarrhoea.

John's problems were now becoming worse. He started experiencing double vision, couldn't see colours properly and couldn't concentrate at school. He was also now pooing himself more often, as he would suddenly need to go to the toilet but couldn't hold it. We stopped the Movicol, which led to an increase in stomach wind and he then started to experience pains in his stomach. He developed serious mouth ulcers, breathlessness and cracks in the corners of his mouth. He resorted to continually eating ice. Then his legs started suddenly to give way.

On 5th February I took him to the local optician to make sure there was nothing seriously wrong with his vision. They could find nothing obvious to explain the double vision and lack of colour.

On 12th February a teacher at John's school noticed him struggling in class with his eyes and he was told to rest. I telephoned his GP as he was obviously getting worse and the GP asked us to get an optician's report. The optician agreed to see him straight away. John had a thorough two-hour eye examination. Since the previous appointment the week before his eyesight had deteriorated and he had developed a loss of field of vision. The optician agreed to write a report the next day (as it was 6 pm by this time) and send it to John's GP.

The next day John was sent home from school as he was so ill. Just as I was leaving to get him our GP phoned to see how he was and I explained I was on my way to get John as he was ill at school. The GP unfortunately couldn't see him that day as he was on a half day. The following day, Valentine's day, John was back in front of his GP who agreed, in principle, to prescribe injections but said he would have to check with the partners first as he didn't want any comeback. John provided more blood to check his B$_{12}$ and the doctor also agreed to other tests that I asked for, including thyroid and vitamin D.

The following day the GP telephoned to say his partners had agreed to start injections of B_{12}. Also some of the blood results were back and his folic acid was now elevated and so his daily tablet was reduced to 400 mg. Unfortunately his iron was still low and also his ferritin levels had dropped slightly so we were told to increase the iron tablets to two a day. His B_{12} was over 400 but they still agreed to try injections. These began on 18th February.

John had an injection on Monday, Wednesday and Friday. And that's when the miracle happened. On the Tuesday following the first injection John woke up happy and singing. The symptoms were still there. On the Thursday John sat talking with us and our friends and on the Friday he was asking for cuddles, which was something he hadn't done for months.

On Monday 25th Feb John was away from home on a residential week. He would not have any B_{12}. During that week his hands started going into spasms and he began to experience pins and needles. On the Thursday night he woke up unable to breathe and shaking – this was spotted by another student and reported to his teacher. On 1st March John's GP rang to say the results for vitamin D had come back as low, so he was to be started on 1000 micrograms daily, to be reviewed in three months.

By Monday 4th March John had still only had three injections and he was back to how he had been, with all of the symptoms present but his tiredness was worse than ever due to the residential week. He received three more injections that week, but did not really see much improvement.

On Monday 11th March we were back at the doctor's who agreed to two more weeks of loading doses, three times a week. By the Wednesday there was an improvement. John's eyes were not blurred and he was happy again. He had his last injection of the first week on the Friday but then by Sunday he was really weak and was having trouble swallowing. He was however playing with his Lego which he hadn't done for months as he had trouble holding the pieces and concentrating.

The second week of his loading doses commenced and, although his eyes began to hurt again by the Thursday, he commented he felt like he had actually slept. He was still very forgetful, which was getting to him, as he found it hard to remember items for school and to revise. On Saturday 23rd March we went away as a family and John had to sleep in the same room as us. He actually slept still and through the night which was unusual as he was always up and down in his bed and really restless during the night. However, the next night he was very restless. The next day he was cross with himself and others.

On Monday 25th March we were back at the doctor's. He was happy with John's progress. John's eyes were a lot better and his stomach was calming down and he was sleeping better though he was still having trouble breathing when he did any exercise, and he was still getting occasional mouth ulcers. Family and friends have all commented how much happier John is and his doctor agreed to inject him weekly for six weeks, but the last few days before his injection he gets tired, starts to eat lots of ice and suffers from tinnitus. He's still on weekly injections.

The major issue here is that parents and teachers are unaware that the symptoms of pernicious anaemia will still be experienced by the sufferer even after treatment has begun and therefore ignorance plays a part in adding to the child's troubles. The usually inflexible nature of the school day further compounds issues, because there is often nothing that can be done to make the provision of education geared to the need of the young person. Think about public examinations. Let's imagine that a teenager hits a wall of symptoms in the early afternoon, yet an important three-hour examination is scheduled for 1 pm. Ideally, the pupil would be able to sit the exam in the morning so that he or she can perform at his or her best. Three issues would prevent this. Firstly, teachers are generally unaware that sufferers have ongoing problems because current thinking among medical professionals is that symptoms disappear once replacement B$_{12}$

injections have begun. Secondly, the pupil may hide his or her symptoms because he or she may be embarrassed by the tiredness and not want to be labelled as lazy. Thirdly, even if the pupil's symptoms were recognised and he or she were not ashamed by the symptoms, there might not be the resources or the will within the school to make the necessary quarantine arrangements that would allow the affected pupil to sit the examination in the morning. That pernicious anaemia can and does mean pupils have special educational needs is not recognised – but it should be.

Veronica's story (from Toronto)

I was a very pale child. So very pale. Every picture I was in I looked sick. People always forced me to drink orange juice to make me un-pale. I like orange juice so it wasn't so bad. I remember being clumsy, having trouble going to the bathroom, having no energy, doing poorly in school, being yelled at because I couldn't keep up. I always had trouble breathing, would sleep a lot. I was the only kid in history who didn't want to go to Disney land because there were too many kids and it looked like a lot of walking that would make me tired.

A trip to the dentist when I was seven to fix a cavity where they used nitrous oxide had me bedridden for a month, but the doctors didn't seem to know what was wrong. Our doctor at the time thought it would be torture to give a little child a blood test, so I never had one done. I got better on my own. Well, as better as I could. I was still pale and tired. My mother complained constantly to our family doctor, but he refused to investigate. (My mother is not well educated and has some learning disabilities, so people often ignore or discredit what she says.) I had anxiety attacks, social anxiety attacks, depression and more. I remember as a child being mad that I existed. I didn't want to live – I hated living and wanted it to end. I used to think these things as a small child. I had no friends. Nobody wanted to be friends with the shy girl who cried too much.

I had life-altering symptoms of pernicious anaemia starting at the age of 12. I would tell the doctor that every time I got my period I was unable to function, I would be bedridden and so tired and sick. I would faint at school and cry and cry. I had very heavy periods. He would pat me on the head and tell me the sob story that 85% of girls had bad premenstrual symptoms. My mother tried to fight with him for me and he accused her of being over protective and neurotic, although recently he apologised to my mother for that since she still has him as a family doctor. I would have loved to see his face when she told him I had pernicious anaemia.

I would talk to my friends about it, and they would tell me about their period woes, but all agreed they were nothing like mine. No one had depression and anxiety symptoms. When I turned 16 I was unable to continue functioning normally. I was so depressed, and I was confused a lot. I had a hard time telling the difference between what was reality and what was a dream. I had memory trouble and thought I was losing my mind. I think my friends thought I was too. My teachers most definitely thought I was and would berate me constantly for being a poor student because they knew I could do better and thought bad of me for not trying. I was an 'A' student when I didn't have bad symptoms. Everybody seems to think the worst of people when they act differently. On a trip overseas with my high school French class that I had looked forward to my whole life, my symptoms went crazy and took me along for the ride. In Madrid, I heard voices. I was scared of everything. By the time we took the train to Paris, I was losing my mind, but I kept quiet and let them think I was lazy and a bitch. My French teacher even called me that to my face. I had to pee every five minutes and spent half the trip learning to say WC in four different languages. I know now, flying can be dangerous for people with anaemia.

I gained weight because I couldn't do gym or continue on the rowing team. I stopped participating in life and graduated high school by the seat of my pants. I continued to slide deeper. If I didn't do hard work, I found I could function better, so I got lazy on purpose and worked at a sit-down job that didn't require mental or physical effort for four years.

I met someone, moved to a new city and started a family. It should have been wonderful. It wasn't. After I had my first child I sank so deep into a bout of depression and anxiety that I seriously considered killing myself. It was at that time that I enrolled in college and determined to use my abilities to better my life, but I couldn't do It. I had stomach pain, joint pain, was always sick and I couldn't be a mom and a student and gave up. My marriage fell apart. He left me because he couldn't deal with me anymore and I had to move in with my father. I went to the doctor and he gave me medicine and the anxiety improved, but I still had attacks that felt like my heart was going to burst and I still lost my temper for no reason, and I was still tired and cranky, but I was somewhat better. I was able to function even better after breastfeeding ended. I was reconciled with my partner, believing the problem was a severe case of postpartum depression. He felt bad for being so quick to jump ship, but who could really blame him? I was batty!

I enrolled in college again, but slowly the symptoms returned. The harder I worked, the more I fell apart. I quit school again and tried to take a slow-paced job, but my fog was so bad it made me really slow. My boss was abusive and even screamed at me because I 'breathed weird'. I didn't know about the 'sighs' being a symptom yet.

I quit when I found out I was going to have a second child. The problems were the same as with the first child except that this time I couldn't walk far or fast and I couldn't eat anything without severe heartburn. Four months after I had given birth I was really pale. I got angry at being useless and dragged my butt through blood tests and back to the doctor's office. He told me I wasn't taking my prenatal vitamin because my B_{12} was low (though I was, because I had heard it should help me with breast feeding, but he wouldn't believe me) and that I had slightly elevated cholesterol and that I was so tired because I was 'fat and lazy and ate too many cookies'. He ignored the low B_{12}, and thought the problem was cholesterol. I left the office in tears. I am a very active person by nature. I can't be active like I want because I am sooooo tired. It hurt to hear. I suffered on.

Breastfeeding was horribly difficult with my second son. He was colicky and if I had known that not having B$_{12}$ was hurting me and him I would have bottle-fed him. I didn't make enough milk and had to pump to make enough to supplement him. I was always pumping just to get enough. That doctor should have known that this was dangerous; he knew I was breastfeeding and he said nothing. I should have known better, but that is the problem with this disease, you just can't think straight! My son is fine now. He got better after eating solid food started. He has sleep apnoea and will be treated for that soon by a paediatrician that I got my children after I started treatment for pernicious anaemia and realised I hadn't been thinking straight. (I don't know if this is important – my mom, dad and I, and my second son, all have (had) a form of sleep apnoea. Not sure if it's related, but I'll put it out there for whoever reads this....)

I got better sometime after breastfeeding was over, but nowhere near what I was before. The fact that I was slow and tired meant that my family just adjusted too. I never really recovered after my second child. I couldn't work. I could barely walk to the bus stop. I couldn't play in the park with my kids. It was easy for me and everyone else to believe that I was so tired because I was fat and I thought it must be that too. I had a friend, though, who was over 200 pounds and she had tons of energy, so I didn't quite think it was my weight, but what could it be? I became reliant on my man to support me and our kids since I was useless.

This next problem is not one I would want to talk about, but since I have to talk about my pernicious anaemia symptoms and if it helps anyone I will, so here it is. I developed very bad haemorrhoids, and while I don't want to talk about my bowel movements, the worst part of this was my digestion. I bled a lot every time I went to the bathroom. I would bleed so much that I started buying gauze and antibiotic cream so I could treat my ass after every movement.

There is a family doctor shortage in Ontario, Canada, so I didn't have a family doctor and would have had to go to the walk-in clinic. After the last clinic doctor called me fat I didn't want to tell them I had this problem, because you can also get haemorrhoids from being overweight.

However, I Googled it and no one talked about amounts of blood like I had. I kept silent.

I had always wanted three children. I tried eating well and forced myself to start working out regardless of how tired I was. Then I was finally pregnant, after eight months of trying, with my third child. During this pregnancy I took my blood tests late in the pregnancy because I was busy moving. Long story short, my landlord was arrested and extradited to the United States on fraud charges and the FBI seized his house, and while they were understanding that I was a tenant, they needed me out of the property fast. I had a lot of distractions during the first part of my pregnancy with this child.

When the results of my blood tests came in the doctor (a different doctor than the 'fat and lazy' guy) called in a panic. I went in that day and he said my B_{12} was so low he couldn't figure out why I wasn't dead. I told him about the test with my second child and he looked at me funny, shrugged and said, 'I've heard of that. Some people just can't get B_{12} in them.' He sent me immediately to the pharmacy and I bought a small vial of B_{12} for five bucks and he gave me a needle and told me to come back in exactly one week. I went home and my arm hurt like mad, but what happened next was the miracle. I woke up in the middle of the night and took a deep breath! I was alive, my senses were so sharp! I felt like a newborn foal! I did grocery shopping and went to the park with the kids in the same day! I had bone pain, deep bone pain so bad that I cried, but my muscle pain was gone! The bone pain went away quickly and I was sooo alive.

The day before I needed the next shot, the muscle pain and fog had returned, but the day after the shot, my life was back to fun!

I tried to tell the doctor at the clinic about it, but there was not enough time to tell them the whole of my life in a short visit, and I was sobbing at the time, trying to tell him he had saved my life. Just one more person to add to the list of people who have thought I was bat shit crazy over the years, but I don't care. I'm not a clutz anymore. I can type fast on the keyboard, I can run, I have started working out again, I don't have hair falling out in giant clumps, I don't have heartburn, I don't have fuzzy feet, I don't have trouble going to the bathroom (I am regular, every morning, on time every time, you could set a clock by it), I am not depressed, I don't have trouble talking to people, the anxiety is gone, I don't see or hear things that aren't there (never really a big problem but now and then I would hear ringing I couldn't explain, or see shadows that weren't there), I can breathe! My tongue isn't fat anymore and I can now do the hotdog tongue trick that all the other kids could do but I never could. My man thinks I'm hilarious because I am discovering all the neat things I can do. My headaches are gone too.

It has been nine months since I first started getting jabbed. My life, every minute of it, I have been enjoying. My new baby is happy and I am happy too. My kids can't believe that I am playing with them. I thought I might be better enough to finish my education and tried and have now completed my first online class. A few more credits and I'll be a college grad! I might get this finished! If I can get my typing speed up, I will be able to get a job. I am excited at the possibility of having a normal life. I am getting housework done at a rate I have never done before. My house is starting to look like other people's houses. I vacuumed and dusted three times this week!

18 to 22 years old

Although not strictly children any more, young adults with pernicious anaemia who are still symptomatic will find the disease affecting not only their higher education but also their social life. In terms of education, their condition will often play a part in their decision whether or not to continue education at all. This will depend, of course, on the way in which they are still experiencing the symptoms of the disease. In the worst cases, they will decide that they will not be able to cope with the demands of higher education, and not continue with formal education or training.

Marie's story

In November 2012 a new volunteer arrived at the Pernicious Anaemia Society's offices. Marie was 22 years old and looking to gain experience of office work. She offered to do two days a week of volunteering. I sat down and discussed what we needed done and how she could help. 'The problem I have is that I have chronic fatigue syndrome and I can't do mornings,' she told me. I was intrigued. I asked how long she had been suffering. 'Oh, I haven't been to school since I was 13,' she told me. 'I just couldn't get up in the mornings or concentrate.' She was the direct opposite of me – I only do mornings! Out of curiosity I asked to see her tongue. It was swollen, red and 'beefy'. I told her that I thought she had B_{12} deficiency, probably caused by pernicious anaemia. She laughed. 'I've seen so many different doctors and given so much blood I would have been bound to have been told if I was,' she told me, reasonably.

Over the next few weeks I became more and more convinced that Marie had B_{12} deficiency. She was not a vegetarian or vegan and she ate a healthy balanced diet. If she did have a B_{12} deficiency it was most likely to be caused by pernicious anaemia.

Christmas arrived and, as in previous years, all of the volunteers descended on a local restaurant to have Christmas Lunch. On the second glass of wine I suggested that Marie might benefit from having a B_{12} test. 'You're obsessed with B_{12},' she told me, probably correctly. An hour later, after I had suggested the same thing again she gave in: 'Alright, alright – you win. I'll arrange to go and see my doctor in the new year.' I told her not to ask for a blood test but to specifically ask for her B_{12} to be checked.[x] The new year arrived, and one morning I had a telephone call from Marie.

'I've just telephoned my surgery for the results of my B_{12} test. You

x B_{12} is not included in the full blood count. Doctors rely on enlarged red blood cells (macrocytosis) to be an indicator of B_{12} deficiency even though a deficiency results in enlarged red blood cells in only around 60% of patients.

were right. My level is 112 pcmol/ml and the threshold to determine deficiency is 190.' I asked when she would have her first injection. Her answer should not have surprised me, but it did.

'They told me to go back in six months and they would check it again, then maybe have an injection.' Following my advice, Marie immediately made an appointment to see her GP and her loading doses began. She has since received an intravenous infusion and is self-injecting every other day. She is now studying for her A-levels by distance learning in an effort to catch up on her missed schooling. She has had an offer of a place at university, dependent upon her A-level results.

Then there are those young people who enrol in a higher education course only to find that they cannot cope with the academic rigour of the subject and have to give up their studies. I have, in the past, helped around half a dozen students to negotiate a teaching programme based on the worst effects of their condition by liaising with their personal tutor. A few times this has not been possible and the student has left the course, often after making huge efforts to meet its demands. One young lady simply changed her study area and enrolled on a completely different course because all of the lectures and classes took place, fortuitously, in the afternoons, she being a morning sufferer. I don't know if it worked out for her as in subsequent years of the course the lectures might have been held in the mornings.

Universities are generally places where the individual needs of students are assessed and met in order to ensure that everyone has equal opportunities to take advantage of higher education or to follow a vocational qualification. They were among the pioneers in ensuring that equal opportunities were afforded everyone regardless of any disability, and the built environment was altered to ensure this was the case. New buildings are now designed to ensure that any physical disability will not be a barrier to a person realising his or her full potential. However, if that student is still symptomatic with the worst effects of pernicious anaemia, then it is not guaranteed that the college concerned will be able to meet his or her needs, often because pernicious anaemia sufferers are not thought to have any special needs as he or she will be receiving what is believed to be adequate B_{12} replacement treatment. We, as a patient group, are still at the bottom of a steep hill when it comes to educating wider society that sufferers can still be symptomatic even after treatment has begun.

Higher education is not just all about learning – it's about interacting with others of the same age and with experts in the chosen field of study. Often it is the first time that the young adult will have left home and he or she will begin to explore the freedoms that come with that. The social side of university life is an integral part of the whole higher education experience, and that doesn't mean spending every waking hour in the Student Union bar. It's about joining and participating in the various student societies. It's about meeting new friends with similar interests. It's about learning more, experiencing more and developing new skills, social or otherwise. I will leave it to the reader to imagine how those who are still experiencing the strange tiredness, the brain fogs, the memory problems and the mood swings will be able to cope with the social side of university life.

Conclusion

In this chapter I have tried to show how the lives of infants, children, adolescents and young adults who have pernicious anaemia and who are still symptomatic will be affected to a greater or lesser degree by the illness. It will affect their education and their social life during a time when personalities and lifestyles are developing and when they should be happiest. While some sufferers will not have their early years affected by the worst effects of pernicious anaemia, others will, and where this is the case it can and does impact on educational attainment and social life. Just as with adults, the way in which the sufferer is able to cope will depend on how much others understand that pernicious anaemia can still be a problem even after treatment has been started to correct the biological aspects of the disease. Hopefully this chapter will have helped to foster that understanding.

Chapter 6

The causes and consequences of pernicious anaemia and vitamin B$_{12}$ deficiency

I experienced nearly all of the common symptoms of pernicious anaemia before being diagnosed. But because those symptoms crept up on me and developed insidiously I attributed them to my having reached 40 years of age. I thought that the constant tiredness, cognitive issues, loss of memory and erratic behaviour could all be due to natural ageing. I had experienced these problems for nearly two years and it was only when my legs went numb that I visited my doctor. I didn't tell him about how I was feeling, how I was having problems with carrying out my duties as a further and higher education teacher – I concentrated solely on my legs. I had had a fall a few weeks earlier and, quite rightly, he associated the numbness with the fall and suggested that we wait a few weeks to see if the feeling came back. If I had mentioned all of my other symptoms he might, just might, have investigated why I was feeling and behaving as I was, and he might have been concerned that my neuropathy (nerve damage) and other symptoms pointed towards sub-acute combined degeneration of the spinal cord secondary to pernicious anaemia. As it happened, it was another nine months before I was eventually to receive a diagnosis but only after I could only walk while holding onto something, and my sister, who is a nurse, decided to take blood. By then it was too late. My central and peripheral nervous systems had been deprived of B$_{12}$ for so long that they had degenerated.

I still have most of the symptoms of pernicious anaemia even though I self-inject highly concentrated B$_{12}$ (in the form of methyl-cobalamin) every other day. I lost my career but cannot blame that on medical professionals. I hadn't considered that the many symptoms that I had been experiencing were all related and I certainly hadn't expected them to be due to a vitamin deficiency. That's why I started the Pernicious Anaemia Society – I wanted to help others like me to understand the condition and maybe, just maybe, raise awareness among wider society and among medical professionals of the symptoms of the disease so that it could be detected before any serious, irreversible nerve damage occurred. What I have inadvertently uncovered is that there are serious problems with the way in which pernicious anaemia is both diagnosed and treated. These problems became evident from the very day the Society's online forum went live and what's more, these issues are not confined to any one country but are worldwide. But why are there such shortfalls in the detection and treatment of pernicious anaemia? Why have these issues not been corrected by medical professionals? And why is nothing being done about it? These are three highly relevant questions to which I will now suggest answers.

The first thing to understand about why these obvious problems have not only developed but lain unresolved is the very nature of patient support groups. They are for patients and do not generally communicate with, or influence, healthcare professionals or policy makers. Patient support groups are invaluable in any modern healthcare system for providing not only information and support to patients who have the relevant medical condition, but also a vectoring point where sufferers can interact with others. This can mean not only a place where coping strategies can be exchanged, but also where any problems, complications and concerns can be aired. That's what happened when the Pernicious Anaemia Society came into being: suddenly, and for the first time, there was a forum where patients could exchange their experiences (which they did and still do) and in the process they highlighted the serious issues with the way in which pernicious anaemia is diagnosed and treated.

When the first online forum went live in 2004 it was the only place where people could exchange ideas, experiences and best practice. Now, there are various other forms of social media which do much the same – just take a look at all of the B_{12} deficiency and pernicious anaemia groups that there are on Facebook. Whilst these various groups are able to provide forums where patients can interact with one another, and where the serious problems with diagnosis and treatment can be identified, they are not set up to communicate these issues with health decision-makers. The Pernicious Anaemia Society is able to do this, and has been doing so for the past four years, but only after becoming a credible patient group in the eyes of the UK's doctors. Obviously, some people with B_{12} deficiency do not encounter any problems with getting a diagnosis, and manage perfectly well on the current, standard treatment; these individuals would have no reason to join the Society as they lead perfectly normal lives free of any symptoms. However, with over 7,000 members signed up in around four years, there are plenty of people within the Society who have experienced at first hand why the diagnosis and treatment of pernicious anaemia need to be thoroughly reviewed and overhauled.

That then is a key reason why health professionals haven't addressed what is, to members of the Pernicious Anaemia Society at least, a serious problem with the way in which perni- cious anaemia in particular, and B_{12} deficiency in general, are diagnosed and treated. Before the Society came into existence there was nowhere where patients could interact with each other and collectively identify problems, and there was no representa- tive organisation that could take these problems to the relevant decision-makers to request change.

In my view, the second reason why problems with diagnosing

and treating pernicious anaemia have not been addressed by medical professionals is that since the 1920s the 'pernicious' part of the disease has become redundant. It was during this decade that the American George Whipple cured induced anaemia in dogs by feeding them liver, and soon after his fellow Americans, George Minot and William Murphy,[xi] discovered that when patients with pernicious anaemia ate large amounts of raw liver daily then they would no longer die. This was because their B$_{12}$ deficiency was corrected, even though B$_{12}$ hadn't yet been identified. (Remember, this deficiency was the reason their red blood cells couldn't marry with any haemoglobin and carry oxygen throughout the body.) There are members of the Pernicious Anaemia Society who remember their grandmothers eating around a kilogramme of raw liver (or sometimes hearts) in order to remain alive. Then in the following decades some of the greatest leaps forwards in haematology took place.

In the late 1920s, Edwin Cohn managed to make a concentrate of liver juice that could be injected into patients. This meant that by this time people who were being diagnosed in time could be kept alive, either by eating large amounts of raw liver or by having concentrated liver juice injected into them. Then, in 1947 the Americans, Mary Shorb and Karl Folkers, along with the Scottish Alexander Todd, isolated and identified vitamin B$_{12}$. In the 1950s, the American Robert B Woodward and the Swiss Albert Eschenmoser led teams of 100 scientists, who took 10 years to produce synthetic B$_{12}$, which led unsurprisingly to a rapid decline in the demand for concentrated liver juice.[xii] Then, in 1956 Oxford University's (and Margaret Thatcher's teacher) Mary Crowfoot identified the chemical structure of B$_{12}$, for which

---

xi Whipple, Minot and Murphy shared the Nobel Prize for Medicine in 1934.
xii Woodward was also responsible for producing artificial quinine, cholesterol, cortisone, strychnine, lysergic acid, reserpine, chlorophyll, cephalosporin and colchicine.

she was awarded the Nobel Prize in 1964. And that was the end of that.

By this time then, cheap, safe artificial B_{12} could be given to patients with pernicious anaemia and it would stop them dying. Medical researchers and practitioners who enjoy a challenge began looking at other diseases and pernicious anaemia was, to a certain extent, 'kicked into the long grass'. There it remained until the Pernicious Anaemia Society picked it up and threw it back onto the field of play. However, just because the ball lay in the long grass did not mean that it was being ignored completely. Some of the finest minds of the 20th and 21st centuries have been steadily trying to understand fully the nature of B_{12}, which continues to fascinate and intrigue a dedicated band of medical professionals and other scientists who have long been aware that B_{12} still has some surprises to reveal. I know of doctors who use B_{12} to treat autism, asthma, back pain, diarrhoea and a long list of other medical conditions. The science behind it hasn't been explained (yet) but thankfully that has not stopped them from helping many thousands of grateful patients. On the other hand, there are scientists and doctors who are content to take artificial B_{12} at face value and use it to treat any B_{12} deficiency, whether caused by pernicious anaemia or not. Because of a dedicated group of doctors and other scientists I predict that in the next few years the full remarkable attributes of the most complex vitamin will become known with startling consequences. Until then, I suppose most doctors will simply regard B_{12} as part of their toolkit and not give a second thought to how important a discovery it was in treating what was a disease with a lethal outcome. (Remember, B_{12} is used to *treat* pernicious anaemia – there is still no cure for the disease.)

I think the third reason why these problems with the diagnosis and treatment of B_{12} deficiency have not been addressed is that until recently nobody tried to make medical professionals aware of the impact on patients. I was recently at a meeting with a professor of Primary Care at a large teaching hospital in the UK. I had managed to arrange the meeting with the help of another doctor who is a great supporter of the Pernicious Anaemia Society. After 30 minutes of my explaining the problems members of the Society face in getting an early diagnosis, she simply exclaimed, 'It's a mess, isn't it?' Similarly, at a meeting with a national clinical director, she held her head in her hands and asked in a way that indicated that she didn't expect an answer, 'How much is this costing?' Any medical professional that I have explained our problems to says the same thing – there is an almighty mess in getting patients with pernicious anaemia quickly and accurately diagnosed and adequately treated. But why are we in this situation? Why is it taking so long for our members to receive a diagnosis? Thankfully there are answers to these questions and it all begins with the test to assess whether a patient with some or all of the symptoms of B_{12} deficiency is clinically deficient in the vitamin.

Justine's story

I have been unwell now for 12 years. I first noticed not feeling right in mid 2001. It was subtle at first. I just felt a lack of energy and lack of enthusiasm for work. I would find it terribly hard to get out of bed and spend all day just waiting to get home so I could get back into bed without eating tea. Over a period of six months I had a bad virus, started a new job where there were a lot of office politics and after three months got made redundant. I found a new job and whilst there the illness became worse. I had pains in my thighs and I would shake uncontrollably and become very weak after very little effort. One day I felt so dreadful I collapsed. My boss put me in a taxi and sent me to the nearest NHS walk-in centre. From that point on things were really bad and more symptoms kept coming all the time. Utter exhaustion and weakness, muscle pain, daily headaches and dizziness were the ones I remember most from this time. By January 2002 I decided I would leave work and London, have a break for a few months and then get a new job. Maybe it was just stress? I knew this was wishful thinking but I had to keep positive.

I moved back to my parents and went to my GP. He organised an MRI scan of my brain, as I was getting so many headaches, and some blood tests. I mentioned that my grandad had had pernicious anaemia so would like my B_{12} tested. He had gone through a nightmare, being told he probably had leukaemia and so told the whole family if we ever got ill to make sure we got our B_{12} tested. I have since found out my B_{12} wasn't tested at this time. Everything else came back normal and I was diagnosed with ME and prescribed anti-depressants as I was told these often help with energy in people with ME.

For the next few years I was unwell, trying to pace myself, trying all kinds of alternative remedies. I was bed- or sofa-bound a large proportion of the time, but was able to walk a bit and even get out and see friends sometimes. The anti-depressants did nothing, but when I said this the doctor just put me on a higher dose. I saw lots of specialists as I was developing new symptoms all the time but they all told me I was fine. I had severe heart palpitations and rapid/abnormal heart rate (which I am now on beta blockers for), severe stomach symptoms, concentration and memory problems, intolerance of light and noise and many others to add to the original symptoms.

During this time I was told my cortisol level was low but I was tested for Addison's disease and all was fine. I also saw a neurologist for my headaches who was concerned as he saw a rash on me that he said was an auto-immune rash. He tested me for lupus, which also came back negative. He said I needed treatment for chronic daily headaches and prescribed me amitriptyline and triptans. After I started on the triptans I began to get horrible symptoms where my head would be swooshing and fizzing inside and occasional episodes where I would get unbearably hot, drip with sweat and start to lose consciousness. This stopped when I came off the anti-depressants and started again a few years later when I was put on tramadol. I have since discovered I was suffering from 'serotonin syndrome', which happens when you are prescribed more than one serotonin-based drug; this is potentially life-threatening so I was lucky to have it only relatively mildly, although it didn't feel mild and every time I had a funny turn I went grey and my parents would be on the verge of calling an ambulance, but I would always recover. I was never monitored whilst on these drugs and the worst thing is they were all drugs I probably never needed to be on anyway.

Two years in it seems I finally had my B$_{12}$ and folate tested. At the time I was told both were fine. I have since found out that 'officially' my B$_{12}$ was fine at 179 but my folate was marked as low.

A year later I was told I was slightly anaemic and put on iron pills. They said this was due to my heavy periods. I took some of the iron pills but they made me feel sick so they switched me to liquid. I have since found out that although my haemoglobin and MCV/MCH [mean corpuscular volume to mean corpuscular haemoglobin] were only slightly low, my ferritin level was actually only 2. I wonder if this should have rung alarm bells – that is, was there a competing megaloblastic anaemia going on? At the same time they told me my white blood cell count was low but they didn't know why. My GP wrote to a haematologist. My GP told me the haematologist had said he couldn't see anything wrong but to keep an eye on it. I have since found out from looking at my medical records that the haematologist actually said I had leucopenia [reduced white blood cell count] and borderline neutropenia [reduced blood neutrophil count] and it might be due to low folate as he noted my folate had been low a couple of years before. He asked my GP to check my B$_{12}$ and folate levels again. I had no idea this was being done but according to my records my B$_{12}$ was 161 (the lower limit being 150). My folate result is blank. I am not sure if this result was never received or if my surgery just hasn't provided it to me with my records.

A year later I was told I was anaemic again (again it turns out my ferritin levels were only 3 even after the iron therapy a year before). I took some pills. It seems from my records I was tested again in May and July, and the anaemia was actually getting worse, although I wasn't told this. After this point my MCV started to rise but now I don't know if it was because the iron-deficient anaemia had been successfully treated or if the B_{12}/folate anaemia was just getting worse, or perhaps both.

After this point, around 2005-2006, maybe due to the iron-deficient anaemia being treated or maybe due to the fact I took some B_{12} sublinguals around this time (one of the many alternative treatments I tried), or maybe because I came off the anti-depressants thereby stopping the serotonin syndrome symptoms, I started to slowly improve. This was five years after first becoming ill. I was still symptomatic and weak some of the time, but I began working part time.

After a couple of years I started heading slowly downhill again until I crashed worse than ever. All my symptoms were much worse than before and I had new symptoms such as severe orthostatic intolerance [problems with standing up], severe balance problems and unbearable chronic pins and needles. During this time I genuinely thought I was dying. It felt as if all my bodily systems were shutting down. I was bed-bound and often unable to move. I couldn't stand any light or noise at all. The curtains were constantly drawn. On a very rare good day I would be able to go out in the car or wheelchair for 15 minutes or so. This would be difficult though, due to the orthostatic intolerance, pain, balance problems and weakness just caused by sitting upright. Even my family thought I was dying.

I managed to get to my GP and explained how terrible I was feeling and that I thought I was dying. He laughed and reassured me that I wasn't. He didn't do any tests or an examination; he told me there was nothing else he could do for me. I also told him that I had developed a sudden allergy to wheat. As soon as I ate it I would sneeze, cough and my eyes would water. I would then have terrible stomach issues for the next 24 hours or so. He said it was one of those things and just to stop eating it. I told him that I had to do something so I was considering trying a clinic which specialised in allergy and environmental medicine. He thought this was a good idea. I knew I would die if someone didn't find out what was wrong with me so I asked my parents if they would consider giving me the couple of thousand pounds they had put away for if I got married so I could use it for private treatment. This was a hard thing to have to do but I knew I had to find out.

I somehow made it to the specialist clinic, although I collapsed when I got there and had to be carried to a bed, where I stayed for a few hours. They organised some tests and gave me a list of basic tests for my GP to do. Their tests showed I had barely any mitochondrial function, which I now know can be caused by a lack of B_{12} and high antibodies to a past Epstein Barr virus infection. My GP did the tests he was asked to do, although he said he shouldn't really do them as I was under the private clinic now. He told me they were all normal and I sent them to the clinic. The clinic wrote to me saying that my MCH was high and they were assuming my GP was testing for B_{12} and folate. I now know my MCV was also on the high side at 100.7, but this was marked as normal. I took this letter to my GP, who said there was no way a high MCH would mean low B_{12}. The MCH would be low if there was a problem with B_{12}. I asked him to do the test anyway as it would put my mind at rest as my grandad had had pernicious anaemia. He agreed under sufferance.

I rang for my results and the receptionist said I needed to speak to my doctor on my next visit. She said I didn't need to make a special appointment. I didn't have a next visit planned and I was too unwell to make an appointment there and then, especially if it sounded like it wasn't urgent. I made one a week or so later. Before I went I found the Pernicious Anaemia Society website and looked at their symptom list. I had every single symptom listed except maybe one. I couldn't believe what I was reading. I had never come across all my symptoms listed so precisely. When I went in, my GP explained I had low B_{12} and folate. He said, 'You're a vegetarian, aren't you?' I said 'No, I never have been.' He looked a bit shocked and confused and apologised for not testing me sooner and gave me an injection and said I would have one a month later and then every three months. He also prescribed me two months' worth of 5 mg folic acid. He said it wasn't pernicious anaemia as I wasn't anaemic (meaning iron-deficient anaemic) but he did say my stomach could not absorb B_{12}. He said that this wouldn't be causing my symptoms and that this basically wasn't a big deal; I still mainly had ME and the B_{12} deficiency was just a minor thing and if we all looked hard enough we would all have a deficiency of something. I said that I wanted to know why I wasn't absorbing and could I have the intrinsic factor test. He said GPs weren't allowed to do that test.

After that first injection my orthostatic intolerance improved dramatically. Everything had been going black every time I stood up; after the jab it only happened occasionally, although I would still feel dizzy. My pins and needles improved a bit and I was able to sit upright for twice as long as before. I had been collapsing in the GP's office before the injection just because I couldn't sit upright in the waiting room. Now I could sit for 10 minutes without feeling I was going to pass out. However, after doing some research online I realised I should be having loading doses of B_{12}. I also found that after a few days I started feeling worse and worse every day. By the time the month was up I felt back to square one. I went back to my GP for the jab a month later. I explained how I felt and asked if I could have loading doses. He said he had never heard of them and that B_{12} was one of the vitamins that is toxic if you have too much and it would be dangerous to give injections every other day. I said that if it was OK with him I would be going to another GP in the surgery for a second opinion as I disagreed with what he was saying. At that he decided to Google B_{12} and then he was sorry, he was wrong. He told me to book in for two weeks of loading doses. I tried taking Jarrow methyl sub-linguals during this time, but I didn't feel any benefit from them really.

I suffered quite badly with the loading doses. Having to attend the GP surgery every other day was hard for me, although the fact I could sit up in a chair now helped enormously. I found the injections very painful and I had bruises, my arm swelled up, I had a rash at the injection site and one nurse even scratched my arm whilst giving one injection. A nurse called in sick one day so I had to have two in a row, which the nurse almost didn't give me as she said it would be dangerous as too much B_{12} is toxic. I said I had spoken to the Pernicious Anaemia Society and they had said it was fine so she gave it to me. Most of the nurses refused to inject anywhere other than the arm as they said it wouldn't absorb anywhere else. One nurse injected my thigh as my arms were so bruised, but wasn't happy about it. Another was more than happy to inject in my buttock.

After this I was told I had to wait three months for an injection and that they never injected more regularly than this. After six days I felt myself deteriorating again. The improvements for me were quite minor as I was so unwell. I only really noticed I had improved when I started going downhill again. I waited 35 days but felt so dreadful I went back to the private clinic in a terrible state and they gave me some methyl sub-cutaneous injections to take home. I was terrified of injecting myself so my sister learnt to do it. I found the methyl didn't seem to work as well, but the clinic had told me to inject only once a week so maybe it wasn't enough.

It was at this point I found out by chance that many of my symptoms might have been caused by serotonin syndrome so I had the utterly awful task of trying to come off tramadol. The withdrawal symptoms were hell and it is probably the hardest thing I have ever had to do. I was so angry that I had been prescribed drugs that clashed, hadn't been monitored and even when I had gone to the GP with new symptoms nothing had been done. Going through this at this point really didn't help. This was the final straw and I decided that my GP's surgery had been utterly in-competent and I needed to change. I also got hold of my medical records at this time, which was when I realised how long I had had this B$_{12}$ issue. I started to believe maybe I had never had ME. I also ordered some hydroxocobalamin online and my sister injected me sub-cutaneously every few days. It was all a bit erratic and I found the sub-cutaneous injections didn't give me the improvement an intra-muscular jab did, but I now think it's because I wasn't having them often enough.

The new surgery agreed to inject me every four weeks for a couple of months. I had a horrible experience when I turned up to the nurse after four weeks and she saw my levels were over 1500 and looked horrified and asked me very sternly who had said I could have an injection as my levels were much too high. I was in tears as I had been counting down the days for this jab, feeling worse and worse. I honestly didn't think I could carry on if I didn't get it. She went and spoke to the doctor, who said I could have it, but I needed to speak to the doctor before I had any more.

I had shingles during this time so I was too unwell to get to my sister for jabs. As soon as I was over that I went up to the private clinic for a methyl infusion. The next day I went back to the doctors. It was a different GP and at first she seemed like all the others, saying my levels were high, which meant I now had good stores in the liver. I had prepared my speech though and explained everything. I said I was lasting about six days before going downhill so she agreed to give me weekly jabs for as long as I needed them and she prescribed me more folic acid. The folic acid gave me a bit of a boost and the weekly injections were slow but sure; for a couple of months I was feeling definite improvements. The only real set back I had was when I had to go 10 days over Christmas. The only weird thing was the GP (despite the fact she was senior partner) told me not to mention at reception that the appointments were for injections. It felt like I was doing something wrong.

However, I started going downhill again for the next couple of months. I was terrified. If this wasn't working what else was wrong? Maybe B_{12} wasn't the answer after all. I asked for more tests. My cortisol came back high which resulted in more tests and a lot of stress. I really was utterly despairing and getting more ill. Also it turned out this GP was retiring. She told me she had discussed the issue with the other GPs and they were totally opposed to the idea of giving me regular jabs. I asked if it was worth bringing the Pernicious Anaemia Society information in but she said they knew about it; they just didn't agree. She taught my boyfriend to inject me and during this process we found out she had been injecting me with a sub-cutaneous needle but doing it directed at the muscle in my arm. She did this because I was finding the intra-muscular needle too painful. I don't think she realised it wouldn't be effective that way. When she prescribed us some B_{12} to inject at home she even asked us not to go to the local pharmacy as he had very strong views about not giving regular B$_{12}$. It felt like we were doing something illegal. She seemed as despairing about their views as I was. As good as this GP was, even she didn't know what the symptoms of B$_{12}$ deficiency were and when I mentioned about my pins and needles she said this wasn't a B$_{12}$ symptom but an ME symptom.

It seems that there is complete lack of knowledge or completely wrong knowledge about all aspects of pernicious anaemia in my experience. I am now of the opinion that I don't want the NHS to be involved in any aspect of my illness as they have proven to be utterly incompetent.

I have also been under the eye clinic at the hospital. I had a squint operated on at the age of five and as I got more ill my vision became more blurred and I suffered from double vision. I've been told that this has come back due to a combination of low B$_{12}$, migraines and migraine medication. I also have problems reading, where the lines and words move around. I have been told this happens with brain damage and for a time I had to use a coloured overlay to read. They didn't say this was caused by the low B$_{12}$ but it only started when I started getting very ill and now I don't need it anymore! The eye clinic have been amazed with how well I am controlling my squint now and have to admit it must be due to the B$_{12}$.

My journey isn't at an end yet, I have had some further hiccups with other health problems but I have realised that the single most important thing for me is getting enough B$_{12}$. I am horrified by writing this story. I have had the years from age 25 to now (37) stolen from me. I gave up my career and the chance of having a family. I have lost most of my friends due to the fact I was ill and they didn't understand. I have struggled for money and had to attend a tribunal in order to claim the benefits I'm entitled to. I got to the point where I thought and hoped I would die in my sleep because I couldn't take the intense pain and sickness anymore. I don't know how long it will take to get better or even if I will completely get better. There was more than one opportunity for this to be picked up years before now as I see from my medical records and yet I was basically left to die as my GP told me he was not able to do anything more for me. I had to spend thousands of pounds on private consultations and tests for them to spot something my GP should have spotted for free. Even now that I know what is wrong, the only way I can get treatment that comes close to helping me is by doing it myself, even though it should be available on the NHS.

I hope I am now finally on track and that many of my symptoms can be reversed. It is a crime that medical professionals know so little about this illness and what they do 'know' is often wrong. I hope I can get some of my life back but I still don't understand why I and so many others have to go through this when we suffer from something that should be so simple and easy to detect and treat.

Problems with diagnosing B$_{12}$ deficiency

For nearly 100 years, B$_{12}$ deficiency and pernicious anaemia were diagnosed without the use of any test. Doctors simply arrived at a diagnosis after listening carefully to the symptoms that the patient was experiencing. Pallor, diarrhoea and tiredness were the main indicators of any deficiency. Today, doctors can rely on science-based tests that show how much B$_{12}$ the patient has in his or her blood. But that test is not automatically used by all doctors; it has to be requested separately and specifically. The first test that doctors use to examine a patient's blood is the full blood count. The full blood count does not evaluate the B$_{12}$ level in the patient's blood – but what it does assess is whether the patient's red blood cells are enlarged – that is, 'macrocytic'. Any enlargement of the red blood cells will lead the doctor to investigate just how much alcohol the patient drinks, as alcohol abuse causes the red blood cells to become enlarged. But there is another possible reason for the enlarged red blood cells – low B$_{12}$. So the full blood count (FBC) doesn't automatically measure the level of B_{12} in the patient's blood, but relies on enlarged red blood cells to indicate the possibility that the patient is deficient in the vitamin. Unfortunately, there is a problem here. Low B_{12} levels do not always lead to the red blood cells becoming enlarged. As William Beck puts it:

> Low serum cobalamin levels in the absence of megaloblastic anemia is also encountered. In a study of 70 consecutive patients with pernicious anemia only 45 (64%) had very low cobalamin levels (i.e. under 100 pg/ml). Anemia was absent in 13 (19%) and macrocytosis was absent in 23 (33%).[17]

And, according to Lindenbaum et al:

> Among 141 consecutive patients with neuro-psychiatric abnormalities due to cobalamin deficiency, we found that 40 (28%) had no anemia or macrocytosis.[18]

This means that the reliance by doctors on enlarged red blood cells to indicate B_{12} deficiency is ill founded. This is further complicated by the UK's National Institute for Health and Clinical Excellence (NICE), whose contradictory guidelines state:

> Tests for vitamin B_{12} deficiency should not be carried out unless a full blood count and mean cell volume show macrocytosis.[19]

There is a further problem with relying on enlarged red blood cells to indicate B_{12} deficiency. If you are taking folic acid as a supplement, then this will prevent your red blood cells becoming enlarged even if you are seriously low in B_{12}. Folic acid is routinely added to flour in North America and this is being considered in the UK and in other countries. Folic acid is also one of the added ingredients in breakfast cereals. This means that you may be taking the equivalent of a supplement without even realising it.

So, the diagnostic pathway that doctors rely on to diagnose B_{12} deficiency is seriously flawed. But let's assume that a doctor automatically asks for B_{12} levels to be examined as well as ordering a full blood count. Unfortunately, there are still further problems. During the 1950s various diagnostic tests were developed and introduced that used microbiologic and radioisotope dilution to measure the patient's B_{12} status. The test used to determine whether that deficiency was caused by pernicious anaemia was named after the American doctor who devised it – Robert Schilling – the Schilling test. That test was used for around 30 years and relied on measuring how much radioactive-labelled B_{12} was being absorbed by the patient; it wasn't without its problems and it wasn't 100% reliable. It was eventually withdrawn due to there being a shortage of laboratories who would manufacture the radioactive B_{12} needed. In the past 10 to 15 years, a new test has been introduced that is a combination of the microbiological and radioisotope dilution test and the Schilling test – the 'combined binding luminescence test' or 'CBLA'. However, this test has been shown to be severely flawed.

Recently there have been studies that show the test is giving false normal results for B_{12} status and for intrinsic factor antibodies. A paper recently published in the highly respected *New England Journal of Medicine* shows that the current test, the test that doctors rely on so heavily to determine the status of B_{12} in patients' blood, is missing between 22% and 35% of patients who have B_{12} deficiency; their test readings show that they have normal levels of B_{12} when in fact they are deficient.[20] I hope you will by now be agreeing that the way in which B_{12} deficiency and pernicious anaemia are diagnosed is 'a mess'.

Problems with diagnosis: the implications

These problems with diagnosing B_{12} deficiency and pernicious anaemia have two broad sets of implications; firstly there are the implications for healthcare providers (such as the UK's NHS), and secondly there are the implications for sufferers and their families and friends.

Take a look at the table below. It shows how long respondents to a survey conducted by the Pernicious Anaemia Society took to be diagnosed.[xiii] Nearly 22% had to wait two years, 19% for five years, and 4% for 10 years. Regrettably, 14% of individuals experienced symptoms for more than 10 years prior to diagnosis.

	2 years	5 years	10 years	10 years +
Length of time taken to be diagnosed	22%	19%	4%	14%

There are two things to note about the figures in the table. Firstly, it more or less corresponds to what I would have expected based on the daily telephone calls that I receive. Secondly, this is an unacceptable situation.

Implications for healthcare providers

This delay in diagnosis has two implications for healthcare providers. It means that patients are suffering needlessly, and in some cases developing serious and irreversible neurological damage due to lack of treatment. Secondly, it is costing money – in all probability an awful lot of money that is taken up by repeated and futile visits to GPs and a variety of specialists. That doesn't take into consideration the cost of any wrongly ordered tests or prescribed medicines.

xiii This was based on 889 responses.

Implications for patients

You can only imagine how angry some of the callers to the office of the Pernicious Anaemia Society are. They are usually angry with their own primary care doctor, and often blame him or her for not giving them an accurate and timely diagnosis. They fully expect that their tales of woe will be met with astonishment by whoever takes their call. Instead, they usually find that I, or one of the other volunteers at the office, will sympathise not only with the patient but with the patient's GP as well. It is then that I have to explain as best I can to someone who finds it hard to believe that his or her problem has been due to a lack of a harmless vitamin that it is not only patients who are being let down by the current way B_{12} deficiency is suspected and investigated; it's not fair on doctors that the technology on which they rely to first suggest and then diagnose B_{12} deficiency is flawed, and that this same problem occurs with determining whether that deficiency is due to pernicious anaemia or not.

There are two main consequences. As the table shows, some patients have to wait years, often many years, before being diagnosed and treated. First, these individuals will have to experience the often debilitating symptoms of B_{12} deficiency for many years and this, as we have seen, leads to problems with careers and at home. These consequences are bad enough, but when you consider the second consequence they become very serious indeed; left undiagnosed and untreated, pernicious anaemia can and does lead to serious and irreversible nerve damage. Ultimately of course, it can lead to a slow and drawn-out death.

What exactly was it like to die from pernicious anaemia? What would the unfortunate patient have felt and experienced? I have come across an account of a middle-aged man whose anaemia proved to be pernicious and whose doctors could only look on helplessly as he battled with the final stages of the disease. Writing in the *Canadian Medical and Surgical Journal* in March 1877, two doctors reported how 'GA' (I shall call him 'George') had suffered as he battled with the pernicious aspect of pernicious anaemia.

George's story

Dr William Gardner (Professor of Medical Jurisprudence at McGill University) and Dr William Osler (Professor of Institutes of Medicine at McGill) were practising physicians in Montreal, Canada. A 52-year-old man 'employed at a spike factory' came to their attention. After losing his two sons, 'George' became, according to his friends, 'weaker and lost colour' and his friends induced him to 'go away for a change of air', which he did. He travelled to Toronto to visit his sister. Unfortunately, the doctors reported that 'After exposure to cold and wet he was seized with an illness, setting in with rigors and attended with cough, bloody sputa, and delirium.' This illness lasted a fortnight, and was called by his medical attendant 'congestion of the lungs'.

'Ever since this illness, he has been gradually growing paler and weaker, and liable during the summers, especially that of 1876, to frequent diarrhoea, never very severe, but rather constant. He would often have in the morning one or two loose motions, and during the day have not further trouble from it.

'The symptoms of which he specially complained were weakness, attacks of shortness of breath, when he walked in the cold air, especially if he faced the wind, and diarrhoea – five or six motions every 24 hours. Notwithstanding these symptoms, he had been attending regularly to his occupation, which, however, did not involve much muscular exertion. At this time the most striking feature of his case was a remarkable waxy pallor of the skin and mucous membrane and a pearly appearance of the white of the eyes.'

The two doctors began to monitor their patient and go on to describe George's symptoms which will sound familiar to most patients with pernicious anaemia: 'Pulse rather more frequent than normal; temperature normal. Appetite by his own account and that of his friends, is good. He is able to eat meat; suffers no distress after food.' They then go on to say that their patient, 'Sleeps very soundly, and sleeps a great deal, much more than previous to the failure of his health. If he sits down and is let alone he is sure to go asleep.'

Then they describe a symptom that regularly crops up in early accounts of pernicious anaemia, but which seems to have been forgotten: George 'is compelled to be up two or three times each night to make water. Urine very highly coloured; quantity in 24 hours is 34 to 40 ounces; specific gravity varied from 1012 to 1016 at different times.'[xiv]

George had also, unfortunately, developed neurological problems as a result of his pernicious anaemia: 'Complains of some numbness of his fingers, hands and forearms; has difficulty in buttoning his clothes, or in using his tools. Complains of a throbbing, rushing sensation in his temples. Says that he has suffered from decided diarrhoea for rather more than a month, but the number of motions in each 24 hours has not exceeded five or six. They have been painless and free of blood...There is a distinct bruit[xv] in the vessels of the neck and upper part of the chest.'

The breathlessness of their patient was also noted: 'The symptom of which he complained most was the shortage of breath, which, as already mentioned, came on when he attempted to walk facing a wind, and was so urgent as to compel him to stop for a minute or two till he recovered his breath.'

The two doctors prescribed Liquor Ferri Pernitratis for George's diarrhoea, but although they had diagnosed him as suffering from pernicious anaemia they had no way of treating him – it would be another 40 years before it was noted that eating large amounts of raw liver could keep patients alive.

George continued to visit the two doctors every week but he was 'growing steadily weaker'. They hadn't seen him for two weeks when,

xiv The specific gravity of urine is analysed to ensure the kidneys are working properly in getting rid of toxins etc. Healthy people's urine will be between 1010 and 1025.
xv Bruit is the term for the unusual sound that blood makes when it rushes past an obstruction.

on 29th December 1876 they received a message asking them to see their patient at his house. They noted: 'There was little change to note in his condition, other than an intensification of the symptoms previously noted. The pallor was more intense, the weakness greater, the drowsiness and deafness more marked, but in addition there was slight oedema of the ankles and eyelids.'[xvi]

George was dying and there was nothing the doctors could do other than prescribe Vallet's pills,[xvii] which were taken for a week 'without the slightest benefit, as he continued to grow steadily weaker and worse, being scarcely able to leave his bed'.

Things got worse: 'On the evening of the 11th January of the present year, an urgent message to see him was received. On reaching his house it was found that on being assisted out of bed to make water, he had had an attack, apparently syncopal[xviii] in its nature, and that at times, especially when left to himself, he was rambling and incoherent. He was very restless; pulse 110, temperature 102°. He had also been vomiting'.

Then again: 'Jan 12th – Noon – Temperature has fallen to 101°. Other symptoms as at last report.'

The two doctors then decided to call for help, which arrived in the form of 'Dr Howard, Professor of Medicine, of McGill University'. Dr Howard 'saw him in consultation at this visit, and fully concurred in the diagnosis'.

'At 10 pm the pulse was 105 and the temperature 97.5°.' By now, poor George was unable to get out of his bed and the doctors noted, 'Retention of urine, requiring the use of a catheter. Urine very high-coloured, red-brown.'

'Jan 13th – 11am – Pulse 98, temperature, 97.3°. Not so restless, still incoherent; vomits everything; catheter has to be introduced regularly.'

George died at 3 am on January 14th.

xvi Oedema is also known as 'dropsy' – a build-up of body fluid in tissue, usually in the ankles and feet.
xvii Pills made up of sulphate of iron and carbonate of sodium, named after the Parisian Dr Vallet.
xviii Syncopal is used to describe fainting or passing out.

It is strange to reflect on how the doctors reacted to George's illness. They had diagnosed him as having pernicious anaemia and they must have known what the outcome would be, yet they, and George's family, persisted in trying to find a cure for his illness. The doctors must have felt just as hopeless as George's family felt desperate.

The report by the two doctors culminates in a long description of the condition of the late spike maker's blood taken 15 hours before he died and also after he had expired. This includes the state of the patient's red blood cells but remember, this was in 1877 and it would take many years for the true nature of pernicious anaemia to be understood fully.

Let's leave the 19th century and be a bit more positive. Imagine a patient today is lucky and receives an early diagnosis of pernicious anaemia. The treatment to correct B_{12} deficiency which poor George was unable to receive will mean that he or she will go on to live a long and happy life without any of the symptoms of pernicious anaemia – right? Well, we have seen in previous chapters how patients still suffer even after any B_{12} deficiency has been identified and ostensibly rectified with injections. There are serious issues with the way in which pernicious anaemia is treated.

Problems with treating pernicious anaemia

It's important to remember that there is no cure for people with classic pernicious anaemia. Instead patients have to rely on injections of artificial B_{12} to keep them alive. It is these injections – or the lack of them – that are by far the most common cause of complaint among sufferers.

There are three different types of replacement-therapy injection available. The most commonly used preparation is

cyanocobalamin.[xix] This is usually prescribed as an injection every month in North America and mainland Europe. Cyanocobalamin is converted by the liver into the derivative **hydroxocobalamin**, then **methylcobalamin** and then, finally, **adenosylcobalamin**. In the UK and Australia, hydroxocobalamin is used, which is supposed to be retained by the patient's body for longer than cyanocobalamin, although the evidence for this is very flimsy. No recent research has been done on this, but a report that appeared in the *British Journal of Haematology* in 1967 said:

> *In every case, serum concentrations of vitamin B$_{12}$ greater than 140 and 100 pg/ml persisted after hydroxocobalamin and cyanocobalamin-zinc tannate for twice as long as after cyanocobalamin.*[21]

However, the authors go on:

> *However, differences between patients were very great, such that the entire trial with the three drugs was completed in 11 months in one case but lasted more than 4 years in another. Variation between patients makes it impossible to anticipate the duration of effect of a single injection of one of these drugs in any patient.*[22]

In other words patients vary and consequently the way in which they retain their B$_{12}$ will depend on the individual. Unfortunately, individuality is not taken into consideration by doctors and most people have to accept the treatment determined by their doctor. This is where the problem with treatment begins. The guidelines that doctors follow for treating pernicious anaemia in the UK are contained in the *British National Formulary* – it's that little book that your doctor refers to when he or she needs to ensure that the treatment for all manner of medical conditions is correct. During

---

xix This is formed around cyanide, but the amount is so small that it is considered harmless.

the 1960s the *BNF* (as it is called for short) used to state that a 1 mg/ml injection of hydroxocobalamin should be administered every month; that was changed to every two months in the 1970s and then to every three months in 1984. So the treatment has become less frequent over the years. And it is the frequency of the injections that remains the most common cause of concern of members of the Pernicious Anaemia Society. Some people manage perfectly well on their three-monthly injections – others don't and experience a return of their symptoms long before their injection is due. When the patient returns to his or her doctor and asks for another injection before the standard three months have elapsed, he or she is usually refused. The best outcome that the patient can hope for here is that the doctor will appreciate that it is impossible to overdose with B_{12} and will willingly sanction more frequent injections. (That's what happened with me, although it was my sister and not the practice nurse who used to administer them to me every three weeks.) Unfortunately this outcome is all too rare and there are a number of consequences when the patient's GP won't prescribe any more frequent injections than recommended in the *BNF* or other guidelines.[xx]

The first consequence will be that the patient will be confused as to why his or her doctor won't listen. The symptoms of pernicious anaemia are quite specific – the strange tiredness, the cognitive impairment, the sighs – and if the patient is beginning to experience these again, then he or she will know that the symptoms are those associated with the pernicious anaemia. The patient will then begin to doubt the compassion of his or her doctor, will keep making requests during repeated visits to the doctor's surgery and in some of the worst cases the whole doctor-patient relationship will break down. If the patient hears of fellow sufferers (via the Pernicious Anaemia Society's forum or other social media) who

---

[xx] In countries where cyanocobalamin is prescribed it is usually given every month.

receive injections from their doctor according to their need, then he or she will become not only frustrated but angry – angry with their physician and angry with the system.

The second consequence of the refusal of some doctors to depart from the standard guidelines is completely unnecessary health inequality, especially as more frequent injections are given willingly if the patient is willing to go outside the NHS in the UK, or other public health systems in some other parts of the world. B_{12} injections are given to farm animals, by the way, without any blood being tested – they are given when the animal starts to show symptoms of deficiency.[xxi]

Why is it that some people with pernicious anaemia need more frequent injections than others? Well, it hasn't been fully explained, but it is probably nothing to do with the total amount of B_{12} in the sufferer's blood. It is more likely due to receptors on the sufferer's cell membranes. Some doctors believe that to correct any B_{12} deficiency the patient will need enormous amounts of B_{12} to be delivered via an intravenous drip as it is only by saturating the body with B_{12} that the cells will be 'woken up'. I am unaware of any research to prove this. What I do know is that this method of treatment works in allowing the patient to be symptom free and that many celebrities undergo this form of treatment on a weekly basis.

These intravenous infusions of B_{12} use the biologically 'active' form of B_{12} – methylcobalamin, which only has to be converted to the final form of B_{12} (adenosylcobalamin) by the patient's body. In a survey of over 1,000 members of the Pernicious Anaemia Society, around 10% of patients use methylcobalamin injections. I inject myself with 5 mg/ml of methylcobalamin every two to three days. Believe it or not, methylcobalamin is not licensed for use in the UK or North America, yet it is used by sufferers and some doctors to treat B_{12} deficiency.

xxi See my earlier book *Pernicious Anaemia: the forgotten disease*, page 64.

This is the third consequence of doctors refusing to treat patients according to their needs – patients will turn to help from alternative sources, which can include buying injections from internet 'pharmacies' (I bought some last year from eBay out of curiosity). Obviously, this is potentially very dangerous and is not recommended. Some sufferers in the UK simply travel to continental Europe where the injections can be bought over the counter in pharmacies. They cost around 50p per vial, although there is some price fluctuation from country to country. Often sufferers will then self-inject without receiving any training, without using new needles for each injection and without any lockable sharps bins (jam jars are the receptacle of choice).

Adele's story

As requested, I am sending you my latest news regarding B_{12} injections.

I have been having my injections every three months for 17 years, and intermittently for 20 years previously, due to living abroad.

This year I had the injection on February 2nd and a blood test on April 18th. On May 5th I 'phoned the doctor's surgery for an appointment and was told by the receptionist I had to wait six months as my blood test showed I had B_{12} overload.

On August 2nd I made another appointment for the injection. On entering the nurse's room she told me crossly that I was told to wait six months. I answered that it was six months since my last one. No, she said, six months from the blood test on April 18th.

I became upset as I was having severe spasms in my hands, causing them to turn and curl inwards. I then asked her if I could see the doctor to which she replied she would have a word with her. She left the room, returned quickly and said that the doctor wanted me to wait and not have the injection yet.

I then made another appointment to see the doctor. On seeing her and telling her I was feeling terribly unwell she ordered more blood tests, putting my symptoms down to other things that might be wrong – not mentioning the pernicious anaemia.

On October 6th I saw the doctor and, after I had sat down, she looked me in the eye and asked me why I hadn't had my injections! I was astounded. I told her I had tried to make the two appointments, but had been turned away and told to wait. She did not comment. She then proceeded to lecture me on how important it was to have them regularly!

I then insisted I have the injection at once and she arranged it. She also prescribed two months of folic acid tablets and a course of calcium and vitamin D.

The worst thing about this debacle has been trying to cope not only with the illness caused by having to wait eight months but also with my part-time job – that is, seven hours a week in accounts. I really do not know how I carried on.

Martyn I do hope this letter is helpful to you as you have been so helpful with your advice to me.

Another consequence of the refusal to acknowledge current treatment is unsatisfactory is that no evaluation has taken place of other delivery methods of replacement B$_{12}$ (see page 122). There is some evidence that oral tablets are as effective as injections of B$_{12}$ in correcting any deficiency,[23] and in some countries, notably Sweden and Canada, oral tablets are now the main way in which people who suffer from pernicious anaemia are treated. However, injections remain the firm favourite method of delivery for patients, and doctors in Canada are reported to be reverting back to injections in response to patients' requests to receive them rather than tablets. Other patients just simply bypass their doctor and buy injections of B$_{12}$ in various forms from alternative sources, including the internet. These indications of patient preference lead me to conclude that any attempt by health providers to make just one form of replacement therapy available – for example, by ruling that oral tablets replace injections – will simply drive the issue underground, with doctors losing the ability to oversee their patients who have pernicious anaemia. Patients should be able to choose their preferred method of treatment – the method that works for them – and not have one particular method forced on them.

There's something going on that doesn't make sense. Why would patients prefer to have what can be painful injections rather than simply swallow a tablet to correct their B_{12} deficiency? Why do patients pay for more frequent injections than those prescribed by their health provider? Why do some patients only find relief from their symptoms when they have intravenous infusions of B_{12} that saturate their body? The questions are many and, thankfully, some medical professionals are addressing these though at the time of writing there are no answers. As I have mentioned already, there are suggestions from some quarters that some patients who have total serum B_{12} well above the levels that are deemed to be sufficient might need more because of what needs to happen at cell level, where the B_{12} molecule actually enters each cell. The idea is that the process isn't happening as it should and that only by saturating the cells' B_{12} *receptors* is the molecule enabled to do what it should. Cell receptors are complex proteins that sit on the outside of each cell and manage the entry of specific substances. Thankfully, we do not need to go any further into the complexity of their nature here, but faulty receptors could be the reason why some patients need more frequent injections than others in order to combat the worst effects of their B_{12} deficiency.

Another researcher is looking at whether some patients need much more frequent injections than others is down to differences in gut bacteria in the small intestine where B_{12} is absorbed, while others believe that the problem is due to the complex biological happenings where the B_{12} and intrinsic factor interact.

The reasons why some people with pernicious anaemia need

more frequent replacement therapy than others remain unknown for the time being, but what I find surprising is that doctors immediately believe that any patient who wants more B_{12} than is usually prescribed must be 'imagining' his or her symptoms, and put the craving down to injections having 'a placebo effect'. Now, this could be the case, but nobody has investigated it. I suppose it is an easier explanation than trying to unravel the mystery using scientific evidence.

There is one more thing I would like to introduce before we move away from the questions surrounding some patients needing more B_{12} than others. It *could* and I use the italics to emphasise this, it could be because the very nature of pernicious anaemia centres around having 'good' days and 'bad' days. Bad days are days when the fogs return along with the strange tiredness and one's other symptoms. These could be due to over-exertion, either physically or mentally, or they could be due to some other unknown factor. What is certain is that a large number of sufferers will report that they have occasional bad days followed by good days. Now, if a sufferer has a bad day and then has an injection (or takes a sub-lingual lozenge, say), and the next day feels fine, that *could* be due to the injection kicking in or, and I'm reluctant to say this as I feel I am letting some sufferers down, it could be because they were due a good day anyway and it was just coincidence that the good day followed the treatment. I am going to leave it at that because it goes against what many patients believe, including me – some patients do need more frequent injections than others to derive any benefit. What is interesting is why patients have 'good' and 'bad' days even though they have seemingly excess B_{12} in their blood. Could it be that we are back to what happens at cell level again.

Chapter 6

Hugh's story

I write to provide you with my experience of life including the awful pernicious anaemia.

I was called into the army in 1943 at the age of 18 years and, after training, finished up in Italy in 1944 in a Royal Artillery Unit. After only a few weeks I was, along with two other of my crew, disabled by a shell burst and finished up in a military hospital in Arezzo, where I was treated for my injuries. As a result of concussion my hearing was totally destroyed, for which I still wear hearing aids in both ears and still receive a War Disability Payment from the army.

Coming back into civilian life after the war I finally became a long-distance lorry driver and managed to pursue that occupation until I retired at the age of 65 years. I am married with a wonderful wife and three sons and three daughters, and many grandchildren, who I greatly appreciate.

In 1950 I went to my family doctor complaining of being inexplicably tired and depressed. I asked for time off work to recover, at which the doctor told me in no uncertain terms that I was not going to be off work being paid sick money as well as my wage from work. I was shattered. Two nights later I bought a bottle of sleeping pills and took them all, unbeknown to my wife, and retired to bed! When I came round I was in hospital, where I was treated for depression and received electric convulsive shock treatment. I was sent home a couple of weeks later feeling no better. In the two years following I insisted on, and received, two brain operations – a lobotomy and a leucotomy – which gave me blackouts afterwards, to control which I had to take medication. I was also at this time found to be suffering from pernicious anaemia, for which I have since been injected with B_{12} every three months!

At the time of writing I still receive these injections, but I don't feel any benefit from them. I can only say that I have been through hell with this illness and received no relief from any medical treatment I have been given. My heart goes out to any fellow sufferers who have this awful complaint.

> I write to you in the forlorn hope that you can offer some degree of hope as I am now 88 years of age and my resistance to my illness is naturally growing weaker. I am somewhat uplifted by the thought that you may be the source of help in some degree and perhaps 'lighten the load'.

New replacement-therapy models

In the past few years there has been a marked increase in new preparations of B_{12} that are based on methods of delivery that do not involve injections or tablets. These new products are aimed at the general public who might want to increase their B_{12} levels significantly. There are two main reasons why there is such a growing market for these products, which may be supply led rather than the result of any increase in demand from the general public.

Firstly, it seems to becoming more recognised that the modern diet in the developed world can lead to deficiency in all kinds of vitamins and minerals and therefore supplementation can only be a good thing.

Secondly, and this is more pertinent for B_{12} supplements, incidents of gastric atrophy increase with age and, as the population of developed countries lives longer, more people will develop the condition. As I explained earlier, atrophy of the stomach lining will prevent B_{12} being absorbed from food naturally; supplementation will therefore be needed to ensure good health.

These new products are usually quite potent preparations that often deliver B_{12} in doses way above the recommended daily allowance and they almost exclusively use methylcobalamin as the preferred type of B_{12}, though I have been unable to find out why this is the case. All of the new preparations utilise membranes in the body that allow the B_{12} to be absorbed into the bloodstream, just as nicotine enters the pipe-smoker's bloodstream via these membranes under the tongue and at the back of the mouth. These new products include sublingual lozenges, drops and sprays; skin patches, including some which sit on the skin behind the ear; ointments (the skin is a membrane); and nasal sprays and drops. Some members of the Pernicious Anaemia Society who cannot get access to the more frequent injections they require, turn to these products to help them reach their next injection. One oral preparation includes a full 1 mg of cyanocobalamin along with decent amounts of folic acid and a substance called NAC (N-acetyl cysteine).

Amazingly, nobody has compared the efficacy of these different delivery methods. If anyone did rise to this challenge, they would first need to define just exactly what they mean by 'efficacy', as this cannot apparently be based on how much B_{12} is in the patient's blood; it would have to take into consideration how patients' symptoms responded to the treatment. We may be back once more to the issue of how cells absorb vitamin B_{12}.

Conclusion

The current tests used to diagnose both B_{12} deficiency and pernicious anaemia are seriously flawed, and there are obvious problems with the one-size-fits-all approach to correcting B_{12} deficiency. However, problems with the way in which pernicious anaemia is diagnosed and treated have, on the whole, not been recognised by the medical profession, though there are some doctors who are aware of issues with the current tests, and some are aware that some patients need more treatment than others.

Generally, it is me and a team of volunteers, taking telephone calls, responding to posts on the online forum of the Pernicious Anaemia Society and answering letters, who are aware of the way in which these shortcomings affect the everyday lives of sufferers.

There are some serious questions that need to be addressed.

These include how many people have pernicious anaemia. In a modern, computerised world this should be a relatively easy question to answer, but because misdiagnosis is rife, and because of the length of time it takes for many people to receive an accurate diagnosis, whatever figures are available almost certainly wouldn't be accurate. It would be impossible to give a precise answer by simply analysing the number of prescriptions written for injections of B$_{12}$ (in the UK) because sufferers regularly bypass the established health route and purchase B$_{12}$ from a variety of other sources.

Just how many patients are there who are being treated for depression, multiple sclerosis, chronic fatigue/myalgic encephalopathy, dementia and a host of other conditions when the real cause of their malaise is B$_{12}$ deficiency? If the results of the Pernicious Anaemia Society's survey are an indicator, then the number of patients being erroneously treated in the UK alone would run into the thousands.

However, all is not lost. The Pernicious Anaemia Society is in a unique position to bring to the attention of physicians the fact that these problems have an enormous impact on some people's lives, on their families and on those they work with. Failing to diagnose pernicious anaemia quickly and accurately, and similarly failing to treat patients according to their needs has enormous cost implications for the healthcare system in particular, and the economy in general, as sufferers often underperform in their work for many years before being diagnosed and then make repeated, and often futile, visits to doctors in the primary and secondary care contexts. Nobody is able to estimate just how much money these problems are costing but it is likely to be in the many millions, if not billions, of pounds annually. Hopefully the next few years should see a renewed interest in getting the disease quickly diagnosed and effectively treated. Hopefully this book will go some way to bring this about.

References

1. Smith D, Refsum H. Do we need to reconsider the desirable blood level of vitamin B_{12}? *Journal of Internal Medicine* 2011; 271(2): 179–182.

2. Carmel, R; Holotranscobalamin: Not Ready for Prime Time. *Clinical Chemistry*; 58:3, 2011

3. Carmel, R and Agrawal, Y P (2012) Failures of Cobalamin Assays in Pernicious Anaemia. *The New England Journal of Medicine*. See also David T. Yang, M.D, Rachel J. Cook, M.D. Spurious Elevations of Vitamin B_{12} with Pernicious Anemia: *New England Journal of Medicine*; 366;18

4. Van Rossum et al: False elevations of vitamin B_{12} in patients with pernicious anemia. *Clinical Chemistry and Laboratory Medicine* 2013-0131.

5. These are taken from a survey of over 1,200 members of the Pernicious Anaemia Society.

6. *ACB News* (The Association for Clinical Biochemistry); Issue 600, April 2013, p. 8. See also http://www.ukneqas-haematinics.org.uk/content/News.asp?id=40

7. Lederle F A. Oral cobalamin for pernicious anemia: back from the verge of extinction. *Journal of the American Geriatrics Society* 1998; 46: 1125–7. Kuzminski A M, Del Giacco E J, Allen R H, Stabler S P, Lindenbaum J. Effective treatment of cobalamin deficiency with oral cobalamin.

Blood 1998; 92: 1191–8. Lederle F A. Oral cobalamin for pernicious anemia. Medicine's best kept secret?. *JAMA* 1991; 265: 94–5. Butler C C, Vidal-Alaball et al. Oral vitamin B$_{12}$ versus intramuscular vitamin B$_{12}$ for vitamin B$_{12}$ deficiency: a systematic review of randomized controlled trials. *Family Practice* 2006; 23(3): 279-85. Epub 2006 Apr 3

8. http://forums.phoenixrising.me/index.php?threads/alternative-ways-of-administering-high-dose-vitamin-b12.9868/

9. Okuda K, Takedatsu H. Absorption of vitamin B$_{12}$ in a rectal suppository. *Experimental Biological Medicine* 1966; 123(2): 504-506.

10. Combe J S. History of a case of anaemia. *Transcripts of the Medico-Chirurgical Society, Edinburgh* 1824; 1: 193-198.

11. There are a great many papers that have been published on psychosis and B$_{12}$, of which this is just one: Pavinda G, Hansen T. Vitamin B$_{12}$ deficiency manifested as psychosis without anemia. *American Journal of Psychiatry* 2000; 157: 660-661.

12. Durand C M S, Brazo P. Dollfus S. Psychiatric manifestations of vitamin B$_{12}$ deficiency: a case report: *Encephale* 2003; 29(6): 560-565. MID: 15029091.

13. Ibid.

14. Ibid.

15. Hooper M V. *Pernicious Anaemia: the forgotten disease.* London: Hammersmith Health Books, 2012: 121.

16. *CMA Journal*/January 24, 1976/Vol. 114 113.

17. Beck W S. Neuropsychiatric consequences of cobalamin deficiency. *Advanced Institute of Medicine* 1991; 36: 33-56.

18. Lindenbaum J, Healton E B, et al. Neuropsychiatric disorders caused by cobalamin deficiency in the absence of anemia or macrocytosis. *New England Journal of Medicine* 1988; 318(26): 1720-1728.

19. http://www.nice.org.uk/usingguidance/donotdorec-ommendations/detail.jsp?action=details&dndid=70

20. Carmel R, Agrawal Y P. Failures of cobalamin assays in pernicious anemia. *New England Journal of Medicine* 2012; 367(4): 266.

21. Tudhope G R, Swan H T, Spray G H. Patient variation in pernicious anaemia, as shown in a clinical trial of cyano-cobalamin, hydroxocobalamin and cyanocobalamin–zinc tannate. *British Journal of Haematology* 1967; 13(2): 216–228.

22. Ibid.

23. Vidal-Aiaball J, Butler C C, Cannings-John R, et al. Oral vitamin B_{12} versus intramuscular vitamin B_{12} for vitamin B_{12} deficiency. *Cochrane Database Systematic Review: The Cochrane Collaboration* 2005; 20(3): CD004655.

Appendix

Useful sources of help

Support groups

Further advice and support can be found by contacting:

The Pernicious Anaemia Society
Level Four
Brackla House
Brackla Street
BRIDGEND
CF31 1BZ
UK
Tel: +44 (0)1656 769717
www.pernicious-anaemia-society.org

The Vitamin B_{12} Deficiency Group
www.b12d.org

Other forms of support can be found on the various B_{12} deficiency and pernicious anaemia pages on Facebook.

Sources of supplements

You should always consult your doctor before taking any supplements to your prescribed medication. Please note that the efficacy of the supplements listed below has not been evaluated in a scientific way.

If you are pregnant, nursing or taking any medications, consult your doctor before use. Discontinue use and consult your doctor if any adverse reactions occur. Be aware that taking supplements will affect any blood tests that you undergo to determine the level of your serum B_{12}, and also remember that you will need good folate status (healthy levels of folic acid) for the B_{12} supplementation to work.

There are a host of bona fide companies selling B_{12}-related supplements in almost every country. Simply entering 'B_{12} supplements' into a search engine will return a large number of sources of the vitamin. One company (yourhealthbasket) offers a 10% discount to members of the Pernicious Anaemia Society. Amazon and eBay both have a wide variety of B_{12} supplements, including skin patches and sublingual drops.

www.yourhealthbasket.co.uk
Unit 1, The Old Applestore
Chantry Farm
Chantry Lane
Boreham
CM3 3AN, UK
Tel: +44 (0)1245905505
yourhealthbasket sells a wide range of B_{12} supplements including sub-lingual lozenges, nasal sprays and sub-lingual drops.

BetterYou Ltd
Unit 5 Chambers Way
Thorncliffe Park
Chapeltown
Sheffield S35 2PH, UK
Tel: Office: +44(0)114 220 2229, Direct Dial: +44(0) 114 220 2236
www.betteryou.uk.com

Betrinac

This new product has been developed based around 1 mg of B_{12} in cyanocobalamin form and also contains folic acid and N-acetylcysteine (NAC), which is an amino acid that increases levels of an important antioxidant, glutathione. Glutathione is the body's natural antioxidant defence. Many patients with pernicious anaemia find that taking NAC helps combat the continual tiredness that they experience.

In the UK, Betrinac can be contacted on 0800 689 9606.

Website: www.betrinac.com

Specialists

There are a number of doctors who provide a comprehensive range of treatments:

The British Society for Ecological Medicine is a society of qualified doctors who practise complementary medicine and who are aware of the importance of adequate B_{12} status. They can be contacted at:

Administrator

BSEM

c/o New Medicine Group

144 Harley St

London W1G 7LE, UK

Or via their website – www.ecomed.org.uk

Dr Manjeet Riar has helped a great many of the members of the Pernicious Anaemia Society and he conducts clinics in Bridgend, South Wales, and at Ashford in Kent. He can be contacted on +44 (0)1656 646815.

Further Reading

Until recently there was a dearth of written material on pernicious anaemia and B_{12} deficiency. This problem has been addressed by Sally Pacholok and Jeffery Stewart's *Could It Be B_{12}? An Epidemic of Misdiagnosis*. (Second edition, 2011, Quill Driver Books, California, ISBN 978-1-884995-69-9). This magnificent work pulls no punches and is a comprehensive overview of the problems caused by B_{12} deficiency being wrongly diagnosed and the consequences for healthcare.

There is also my first book, to which this is a companion: *Pernicious Anaemia: the forgotten disease*, also published by Hammersmith Health Books.

Index

Note: Footnotes are denoted by the letter n after a page number. The abbreviation PA has been used for pernicious anaemia.

Note: Footnotes are denoted by the letter n after a page number. The abbreviation PA has been used for pernicious anaemia.

Note: Footnotes are denoted by the letter n after a page number. The abbreviation PA has been used for pernicious anaemia.

Note: Footnotes are denoted by the letter n after a page number. The abbreviation PA has been used for pernicious anaemia.

Note: Footnotes are denoted by the letter n after a page number. The abbreviation PA has been used for pernicious anaemia.

Note: Footnotes are denoted by the letter n after a page number. The abbreviation PA has been used for pernicious anaemia.

Note: Footnotes are denoted by the letter n after a page number. The abbreviation PA has been used for pernicious anaemia.

Note: Footnotes are denoted by the letter n after a page number. The abbreviation PA has been used for pernicious anaemia.

Index

Note: Footnotes are denoted by the letter n after a page number. The abbreviation PA has been used for pernicious anaemia.